THE CAREGIVERS

*A Support Group's Stories
of Slow Loss, Courage, and Love*

NELL LAKE

SCRIBNER

New York   London   Toronto   Sydney   New Delhi

SCRIBNER
A Division of Simon & Schuster, Inc.
1230 Avenue of the Americas
New York, NY 10020

First Scribner hardcover edition February 2014

SCRIBNER and design are registered trademarks of The Gale Group, Inc.,
used under license by Simon & Schuster, Inc., the publisher of this work.

For information about special discounts for bulk purchases,
please contact Simon & Schuster Special Sales at 1-866-506-1949
or business@simonandschuster.com.

The Simon & Schuster Speakers Bureau can bring authors to your live event.
For more information or to book an event contact the Simon & Schuster Speakers Bureau
at 1-866-248-3049 or visit our website at www.simonspeakers.com.

Manufactured in the United States of America

1   3   5   7   9   10   8   6   4   2

Library of Congress Control Number: 2013037357

ISBN 978-1-4516-7414-9
ISBN 978-1-4516-7416-3 (ebook)

For Antonia Lake and Anthony Lake,
who taught me to care,

and for Doug, Galen, and Jordan Winsor,
who help me remember.

That time of year thou mayst in me behold
When yellow leaves, or none, or few, do hang
Upon those boughs which shake against the cold,
Bare ruin'd choirs, where late the sweet birds sang.
In me thou see'st the twilight of such day
As after sunset fadeth in the west,
Which by and by black night doth take away,
Death's second self, that seals up all in rest.
In me thou see'st the glowing of such fire
That on the ashes of his youth doth lie,
As the death-bed whereon it must expire
Consumed with that which it was nourish'd by.
   This thou perceiv'st, which makes thy love more strong,
   To love that well which thou must leave ere long.

—WILLIAM SHAKESPEARE, SONNET 73

CONTENTS

THE CAREGIVERS

PROLOGUE

I remember my grandmother Hildegard—tall, slim-framed, her cardigan and shoes sensible but not quite grandmotherly. She was too stylish for that—wallabies, we called those shoes in the 1970s. In a modernist armchair in her study, listening to NPR, she puffed on a pipe—a pipe! My mother's mother, Hildegard was elegant, German, unadorned, restrained. She had a wide face, high cheekbones, and a gently aquiline nose. I do not remember her embracing me ever; I don't remember sitting in her lap. I do remember the chocolate chip cookies she baked me. She pulled a tin of them from her freezer, layers separated by sheets of wax paper. She held the opened box for me, and I chose one. Cold and hard, loaded with oats and butter, the cookie melted and sweetened in my mouth. She closed the tin.

She strode a mile every day to the center of Litchfield, her Connecticut town, past white clapboard houses with picket fences, and fetched her mail at the post office. She stood by the waste bin and sorted out junk mail. She opened appeals from Planned Parenthood and the Sierra Club and mailed off checks on the spot.

She had filled her big laundry room with supplies for her orderly, practical, and beautiful life: rakes and edge trimmers, bleach and soap, wooden drying racks, winter hats and gloves, seeds and pots. I remember my voice echoing against the walls. She scooped kibble from a drum to a dish she'd set on the concrete floor. Her leggy poodle, Justin, gobbled and wagged. She allowed no dust.

I smelled lavender in the sunny upstairs bathroom, and glycerin soap in a stainless steel dish, and the clean sodium of her tooth powder. My cousin and I, when we were ten, lived with her for a summer week. In my grandmother's bedroom, my cousin and I did *not* jump on the single beds, covered in white, made up tightly. We cleared our dishes away after meals; we played on our own. On steamy days I dipped my hands into the ceramic birdbath my grandmother had placed below the rhododendrons. She'd cultivated native ground covers in the small woods behind the house and left much of the lawn long, in silver and green grasses. She'd had the gardener mow a winding path through the grass toward the vegetable garden in back, where she grew raspberries. My cousin and I ran down the swerving trail and plucked fruit. Our fingers smeared red juice on our cheeks.

My grandmother prized independence and physical vitality. During the time I knew her, she expressed aversion to growing old, particularly to ending up frail in a nursing home. She was uncomfortable with decline and vulnerability, her own and others'. She kept brochures from the Hemlock Society—the pioneering "death with dignity" organization—in a kitchen drawer.

At seventy-eight, in August of my nineteenth year, she learned from a doctor that pain she'd been feeling in her back could mean cancer. She needed tests. That same night, in the garage next to the immaculate laundry room, she turned on the car. The next day, an elderly neighbor discovered her.

It's clear to me that, by committing suicide, my grandmother wanted to avoid being an invalid, dependent. It also seems clear that she didn't want to be cared for. My parents and cousins and aunts and uncles reminded one another of this. Still, I've puzzled, since then, over her death. I've realized not only the ambiguities of my grandmother's last act, but what she subsequently missed—what *I* missed: the intimacy that may come with tending and being tended to. The opportunity to love, to move toward even what frightens us. Perhaps she ducked out to evade the inevitable closeness, the letting go, the being known, the not knowing.

I know well her essential ethic; it has been passed down, in milder form, to me. A worthwhile life, according to my female forebears, is physically vital and wholesome—active, creative, replete with good cheer and fresh air. My mother, sister, and I savor our vegetable gardens and long hikes and thrown pottery and hand-knit mittens. We attend to homey detail, clear the clutter off counters, and fill our houses with color. We hang laundry on lines because wind and sunshine make the clothes smell best. The sight of white sheets on a bright June day, against blue sky and new green leaves, is good for the soul.

Such physical wholesomeness and beauty feel akin to dignity, grace. Hildegard lived this. She also greatly feared its shadow: the fading of the light, declining vigor, the decay, the messiness of illness and dying. What this meant fundamentally, I think, was that she feared losing control.

My grandmother's conscious fear of the shadow part of life may not have been typical. But because I inherited a similar uneasiness with matters of illness and dying, it's fitting, if perhaps not fated, that, twenty-five years after her suicide, I found myself, by happenstance at first, immersed in the lives of a group of people living in that shadow: the members of a support group for women and men tending family members with dementia and other chronic illnesses. In late 2009, I'd attended a birthday dinner for a friend and ended up seated next to one Benjamin Cooper. He told me he worked as a counselor at a local hospital, and that he facilitated a support group for family caregivers. I replied that I was a journalist interested in health, mental health, and medicine. Ben invited me to sit in on his group, as he thought their stories were important and illustrated challenges that more and more people face.

He asked the group members' permissions, and they welcomed me. They knew similar groups were becoming more common. They seemed eager for recognition of their experiences and said they wanted me to listen, to witness. They said that their support group gave them the solace of intimate, relevant stories. They hoped, generously, that an account of their experiences would help others. Soon I accompanied them in their daily lives, becoming privy to inner and outer dramas—the setbacks, the near-deaths and deaths, the anger and perseverance.

It didn't take long before my outlook widened, and my role as well: If I started as a distanced journalist, I became some hybrid—detached writer still, when I could manage it, but also friend and, sometimes, helper to the people I write about here. The shift was unavoidable from the time they welcomed me as a member of the group. I grew to care a great deal about my subjects. Along the way, I drew closer to what my grandmother had fled.

My focus was on the caregivers' personal challenges. But as Ben had said, they *were* living out pressing public-health issues, questions our society needs to address: How will we respond to—and pay for—the fast-expanding need for elder care? How can we tend to the aging, ill, and dying with skill and compassion, while guarding the time, sanity, and finances of the family members who do the tending?

It is a modern conundrum. People used to die far more quickly. Medical advances have wrought a paradox: We're surviving longer, but spending more of our late lives in drawn-out illness, dying protracted deaths. While life expectancy has increased, so too has chronic disease. The statistics show it clearly: More than a third of elderly men and a quarter of elderly women report having heart disease. Half of the old have high blood pressure, and a quarter have cancer. Many with chronic disease stay alive through interventions that did not exist even a few decades ago. More and more are becoming "old old," spending their final years ill and/or frail and unable to care for themselves.

At least in part because of increased longevity, more people are developing dementia—a gradually progressive, incurable impairment of memory, reasoning, language, and personality, caused by one or more brain diseases such as Alzheimer's. Dementia is a central and frightening specter of old age because it slowly diminishes personhood itself and devastates the relationships that personhood enables. With dementia care, children reverse roles with parents; spouses lose partners while they're still around. More than 5 million people have Alzheimer's, the most common form of dementia. By 2050, this number is likely to nearly triple. One in three elderly have Alzheimer's or another form of dementia when he or she dies.

With this increase in chronic disease, more and more people depend each year on day-to-day care from family members and friends. The demand for unpaid, at-home care is accelerating as baby boomers age and the health care system is stretched thin. A few statistics here give a sense for the number of lives affected: According to the Family Caregiver Alliance, more than 43 million Americans—about 18 percent of adults—tend a family member or friend who is older than fifty. Dementia caregivers make up about a third of them. Informal caregivers are the largest source of long-term care in the United States, contributing labor worth nearly half a trillion dollars. Health scholars expect that by 2050, the demand for long-term care will nearly double, and family caregivers will continue to meet the greatest part of that need. Seventeen percent of employed Americans look after an elderly family member; a tenth of these caregivers quit their jobs to provide full-time care, losing potential health insurance benefits and, on average, more than $300,000 in lifetime wages, Social Security, and pension income.

Americans use the word *caregiver* to describe roles that are formal and informal, paid and unpaid. I write here about the latter type: people who give care out of love and/or a sense of obligation. Informal caregivers face fairly universal challenges: emotional and financial strain, physical stress and exhaustion. The particular caregivers I followed endured these difficulties and felt the strains. Caregivers in general experience greater stress and illness, and die at higher rates, than non-caregivers.

Penny, a central figure in this book, is statistically typical of such informal caregivers—a middle-aged, white, employed woman who spends about twenty hours a week caring directly for her mother. The members of the support group I followed weren't, however, altogether demographically average. More of them were elderly, and more were tending spouses (as opposed to parents) than is typical. The group had relatively few caregivers who were parenting young children, likely because people in this situation have the least time for attending support groups. The caregivers were all white and obviously did not represent the racial diversity of this country. Finally, the group members were relatively stable financially—more secure than many Americans. But for them, as for virtually all caregivers, the financial costs of care caused strain.

Within the world that such statistics seek to describe, caregivers' personal lives unfold. Sitting in on the group, I felt I was witnessing a sort of necessary, intimate, private heroism. The caregivers stood face-to-face with cruel decline, with hard choices, with no choices at all. Early on, while attending the meetings, I was moved by this. I also felt affronted. I found it difficult to stay open to their struggles—not just to their suffering, but to what seemed like a fundamental injustice: People we love can disassemble, can descend into oblivion without apparent reason. They suffer, and the people who love them suffer. Their vitality—and in the case of dementia, their essential selfhood—fades. Caregivers must tolerate, and persevere through, disintegration. The support-group members wrestled with a basic fact of our human condition: none of us and nothing lasts. In the bland conference room of a local hospital, ordinary people faced the inconvenient, heartbreaking, and inescapable truth that the body declines, that the mind can fade, that a person we thought was fixed, solid, stable—slowly, inexorably dissolves.

And by extension: we will cease, too—slowly, suddenly, or in some manner in between.

A few in my family held my grandmother's death as a heroic tale of taking control of one's fate, of refusing to be helpless. I can see it this way. But it seems mostly a sadder story: it represents, to me, the extreme of my own, my family's, and our larger culture's fear, even terror, of decline, illness, incapacity, dying. Such fear is natural. But the greater the aversion, the more acute the suffering, the less able we are to respond openly, wisely, to our own and others' real lives.

I've come to see that wisdom happens in finding a balance between control and surrender. Sitting in with the support group, I witnessed both a wholesome desire to take charge and make things better, and a necessary acceptance of the stark truth that control, in the end, is elusive. In continually facing what came along—all the surprises, difficulties, and losses—the caregivers grew in wisdom. They also showed great and ordinary courage.

PART I

WINTER

Storms

🌿 Penny

In February 2010, Penny Jessup stands and chats in falling snow, on the campus of the liberal-arts college where she works. Fat flakes tumble down through still air onto Penny's maroon hat, her light-brown bangs, and steel-rimmed, rectangular glasses. Penny and I have just eaten lunch at the college's student center. Over her shoulder I see the campus's ice-covered pond, rimmed by black and leafless trees. On a slope above the pond, closer by, stand the college's greenhouses. Built in the nineteenth century, they are enormous, beautiful boxes of glass, their frames white and ornately Victorian. Inside, palms, orchids, cacti, succulents, citrus, and ferns thrive in controlled temperatures. Whole and separate climates exist side by side: one room is hot and steamy; another, sweet-scented and warm; a third, arid and cool.

Through falling snow, I spy palm leaves clamoring for space inside a high and vaulted glass roof.

I mention Penny's job title.

"You've got to say it in God's voice," she says with a smirk, dropping her voice an octave. *"Manager of Living Collections,"* she booms.

She laughs and heads off to the greenhouses, back to work.

Penny Jessup has, in fact, two jobs. For one she has a godlike

11

title and is paid a salary: she manages a database that keeps track of the ten thousand plants—trees, shrubs, ferns, perennials, succulents, herbs, ground covers, and so on—that live on the college's campus. It's a dream job. "I'm a plant nerd," she says. She *knows* plants, their taxonomy—the families, genera, and species—and throws around Latin plant names the way sports fans pull up baseball rosters in their heads, with playfulness and reverence. Like most sports fans, Penny doesn't just enjoy the names and stats, she loves the things themselves. Most people walk around the college's campus and see texture, color, vistas. Penny sees all that, plus plant types and histories.

Penny's other job is unpaid and has no official title—but if it had, its name would be as godlike as the other. Penny manages the life and care of her forgetful mother, Mary. She gives Mary food, safe shelter, and medications and keeps her mother alive. She often tries to help Mary thrive. Over the coming year, Penny will wrestle with what, exactly, thriving looks like for a woman of eighty-seven who wants only to eat, sleep, watch television, and have occasional, lighthearted conversations with her daughter. Sometimes Penny thinks, Well, what's wrong with that? Other times she worries, As a caregiver, am I doing enough?

This job is so different from keeping plant records. This second job—for which she is not trained—is sad, frustrating, lonely. It is more challenging than the first, even if things so far aren't nearly as bad as they could grow to be—nor as they are, Penny knows, for others in her caregivers support group, and still others all over the country and the world tending to their elderly. Penny's days tick along, in and out of months and seasons, Penny navigating slow loss and the ordinary, maddening frustrations of a life largely given over to someone else's needs.

• • •

One night that same February—in the early hours of what would turn out to be an otherwise unremarkable day for Penny—a storm moves through from the south and unloads six inches of wet, heavy snow on the small city where she lives. Her alarm sounds at six. She pads down the hall, past a second bedroom, where Mary sleeps. As the light rises, Penny shovels her driveway, heaving sloppy scoops onto the yard. After an hour she steps into Mary's room, singing an improvised tune: "Wake up, sleeping beauty." Mary hauls herself up from bed, silver hair tousled. As usual, Penny offers Mary a glass of water and holds out pills for her to swallow: one omeprazole to prevent a recurrence of the bleeding ulcer Mary suffered five years earlier; one Levothyroxine, for hypothyroidism; an iron pill; and an Aricept, which a doctor hopes will stem the symptoms of Mary's deteriorating brain.

Penny kisses her mother five times on the cheek, a practice resurrected from Penny's childhood—except back then the kisses were passed between Mary and Penny's father. Penny hugs her mother, and Mary sighs and lets herself back down onto the bed. Penny softly pounds Mary's back, rear, and legs—"That's just to wake her up more, you know?" Penny explains later—and heads back down the hall. Mary stays in bed, dozing. She won't get up until the home health aide rings the doorbell at nine. Penny gets in her little SUV with two hundred thousand miles on it and drives the two-lane road that runs along the river from Penny's neighborhood to the college town, munching toast with melted cheese, peering through her glasses at the shrouds of white, cementlike snow on contorted branches. Limbs have snapped everywhere.

She arrives at the botanical gardens before most of her colleagues. Tom, one of the gardeners, is the only other staff person there. He appears in the doorway to Penny's office. "Did you see the beech?" he asks. "The one by the fountain?"

"No," she says.

"It's bad."

Penny searches with Tom in closets and cabinets and finds yellow plastic ribbon with CAUTION written along it. She pulls on her coat and follows Tom outside, past snow-covered perennial beds toward the science building. Penny and Tom stop, their way blocked by the sprawling branches of the once-soaring seventy-three-year-old beech. The snow has crushed much of the tree—"as if it had exploded," Tom will later recall. Two opposing limbs have snapped and span low over the gardens. Finer branches rest on the ground, like hands bearing the weight of the limbs.

The beech had been massive, had seemed a protective, nurturing presence. Its trunk was muscular, nearly four feet thick, with bark like the skin of an elephant. Just the day before, the tree had arched over a small tile patio and a fountain. In the fountain's large stone basin stands a snowcapped statue of a young woman, built in memory of a student who died of typhoid fever one hundred years ago. The woman wears a flowing frock, her long hair falling down her back. A plaque at the base of the pool says IN MEMORY OF A BEAUTIFUL LIFE. It is a fitting eulogy for the day—several other old, magnificent trees on the campus have been felled by the storm.

But Penny has her back to the statue and gazes at the tree.

"They're going to have to take it all down," Penny will tell her caregivers support group the next day of the old and sheltering beech. "It's a shame. In the summer it gave good shade."

Tom drapes the tree with yellow ribbon, lest students approach it. Back inside, Penny's day continues as usual. A dual track runs in her mind: her paid job's tasks keep her busy, but she is simultaneously aware of her mother's day, proceeding in her house a few miles to the south. Wednesday's home health aide, Pilar, arriving for her usual nine o'clock appointment—or likely late because of the snow. Mary, hair mussed, roused by the doorbell, getting out of bed, grabbing her royal-blue, four-wheeled walker with its padded seat and carrying basket underneath, rocking down the hall in her nightgown, opening the door and letting Pilar in. Pilar helping Mary shower, frying Mary an egg and setting it with toast on the kitchen table. Mary eating, and Pilar making Mary's double bed, placing the shower chair back in the tub. Pilar returning to the kitchen and watching Mary take the "breakfast meds" out of the organizer on the table and swallowing them. More pills: Namenda, like the Aricept, in the hope that it will help Mary think more clearly; enalapril, for high blood pressure; citalopram, for depression; and two fish oil capsules. Mary dropping herself into her spot on the worn couch in the living room and Pilar turning on the television. Pilar offering to take Mary for a walk, but Mary, as usual, refusing. Today with the snow, Pilar likely doesn't insist (and, Penny confesses, she doesn't know how often Pilar gets Mary walking even when the weather is good). At ten o'clock Pilar will leave, with Mary watching *Family Feud* and later staring at *The Price Is Right.*

As the day wears on, Penny knows the television is still running at her house. About the time Penny starts thinking about breaking for lunch, she can reliably imagine Mary peeling a banana, opening a cup of pudding, perhaps microwaving frozen home-made soup that Penny has left to thaw in the refrigerator. Mary placing her lunch on the seat of her walker, pushing it back to the couch, sitting, and eating off the walker's seat—television still playing. (And perhaps, Penny thinks, creating new stains on the couch and fresh crumbs on the floor.) Getting up later to leave the pudding container and dishes on the counter, and sitting again on the couch. Through the afternoon, gazing at *Who Wants to Be a Millionaire,* and later managing, by clicking around, to switch the channel to TV Land and *Andy Griffith, I Love Lucy, M*A*S*H.*

Mary leaves the couch only to get her lunch, use the bathroom, answer the phone (Penny calls in the middle of each day to check in, but otherwise the phone rarely rings), and, when dark comes, turn on a single light near the television set, a lamp that

John, her late husband, Penny's father, made decades before from an old-fashioned water pump.

Every caregiving story springs from a particular life, spins out from chapters that came before. Penny's is a tale of redemption. Five years earlier, her life had not been going well. She was living in Wisconsin, where she'd earned her master's degree in botany. She'd stayed on and worked for the same university from which she'd gotten her degree, managing collections for its botanic garden. She bought a house. Despite these signs of success, she says, "My life was starting to look like a *Jerry Springer* show." She had a "crazy alcoholic boyfriend," who, she says, tried to control her. "He was a lot of fun. But, man, did he have a temper. I think he was probably an abuser. I don't think it would have ended well." Meanwhile, for most of her adult life she'd been drinking too much, smoking too much marijuana. The drinking made her sick. She had been in the hospital for alcohol poisoning twice before she reached legal drinking age, and a few times after. She saw a doctor after one hospitalization in Wisconsin. "He said, 'Penny, if you *know* you're going to get sick, and you still drink, that's pathological.'"

Telling me this story over lunch, she narrows her hazel eyes. "I thought, 'Hmm, I think I know what *pathological* means.'" She chuckles in a self-effacing way. "'I think it means you're *sick*.' I went home and looked it up. It does. It means you're *sick*." But knowing this, she says, "didn't make a difference for another couple of years." During those years, she was involved with another man who provided her with marijuana. "I'd say, 'I'm only going out with you because you always have pot. And he'd be like, 'That's *okay*!' And I was like, 'This *is* sick.'"

Over the years she said to herself, "I'm going to quit one," the pot or the alcohol. And then: "'No, I'm going to quit the other.

No, I'm going to quit the *other*.' I would *never fathom* quitting both at the same time. I had to have something to numb me out." Looking back, she thinks she functioned well, despite the troubles with chemicals. But she had other markers of addiction—notably, she says, self-centeredness. She had a hard time getting along with people at her job, offered her opinions freely. "I thought I was providing a public service," she says, laughing. After ten years at her job, she was laid off. She did some consulting for a land conservation group and started a landscaping company—she was freelancing, "aka, hand-to-mouthing it." She broke up with the "crazy, alcoholic boyfriend," which is what she always calls him now, in retrospect.

Then in March 2005, her father passed away, and everything changed. She was at the hospital with him when he died. She remembers her mother crying, her brother sobbing. "I didn't cry," she says. "I was a rock the whole time. It was very strange."

Her parents had long asked, "When are you coming back home?" They and the rest of Penny's four siblings all lived in Connecticut: a schoolteacher, a salesman, a customer-service worker, and a tradesman. After John Jessup's death, Mary's queries became more plaintive: "Will ya come back *now*?" Penny and her sister Sophie talked. Their mother was eighty-two, had struggled to look after their father during his long and varied illnesses. Penny said she'd move home and in with Mary. It seemed like the right thing to do—not just for Mary, but for Penny. She had a place to go.

The decision offered more than cheap housing. In August, a few weeks before she packed up her stuff and headed east, she called her pot-supplying friend for one last party. "Come on over," she said. "We're going to finish my beer. Bring some smokables." The next day she attended her first AA meeting. "I knew that my life had to change. I was going to have to be responsible." She was forty-four. She has not drunk or used pot since, she says. She goes to AA meetings several days a week and "works the program," as AA calls making one's way through the Twelve Steps. She's trying to be less self-centered.

Which isn't to say the struggle is over.

She moved into the red clapboard bungalow she had grown up in. She applied for and was offered her dream job at the college in Massachusetts. She started commuting forty-five minutes each way. She soon noticed Mary was changing. Penny had known that her mother needed her, but wasn't anticipating the extent to which that need would grow. "I thought we were going to be roommates," that living together would be "fun." As best she can remember, the first time she detected something was wrong was when she and Mary were watching a rerun of *House* they'd both seen before. Penny said something about what was going to happen in the story, and Mary said, "How do you know?"

"We've seen it before, Mom."

"I haven't."

"Yes, you have," Penny said.

A few years later she'd try to refrain from such corrections. Honesty, she'd learn in her caregivers support group, is not always the best policy. The theme would become a recurring one for the group—how to roll with your charges' declines, not argue with their misperceptions. A compassionate ideal, hard to practice. You want to say to the husband, wife, mother, you've known for so long, What do you *mean* you can't remember? Where did you *go*? Who *are* you now?

Penny attended a workshop at the college on caring for aging family members. A "geriatric care manager"—a new term for Penny—reviewed health issues among the elderly. Penny raised her hand and said, "I think my mother has a little dementia."

"There's no such thing as having a 'little' dementia," the woman said. "That's sort of like being a little pregnant."

Penny drove her mother for an MRI. They met later with a neurologist. "He was a good neurologist," Penny recalls, "but he had a terrible bedside manner."

"Your brain is shrinking," he said to Mary.

"What can we do?" Penny asked him. In her mind, *brain shrinking* equaled a health problem, and health problems have solutions, or at least partial ones—don't they?

"You can take fish oil," the neurologist said. "But that's not standard of care."

"What would you do if this was your mom?" Penny asked.

"I'd give her the fish oil."

Three years after Penny returned home to Connecticut, she and Mary moved to a town closer to Penny's job. Penny Jessup had become her mother's caregiver, and her care manager—and a keeper of memory. Memories of Penny's childhood and of her mother color Penny's days. The memories aren't always happy, but they aren't dull, either. Her mother loved music, classical mostly. But when Penny's brother brought home *Led Zeppelin III* in the early seventies, Mary blasted the album through the house. Mary played practical jokes on her kids. One April Fools' Day, she sewed the inner tops of their jacket sleeves shut and hung the coats on the newel. "Bus is here! Let's go!" she called. The kids scrambled down the stairs, grabbed their coats, tried to thrust their arms into sleeves. "Come on! Come on!" Mary chided. "You're going to be late!"

Penny laughs, telling me the story.

But even funny family memories can evoke mixed feelings. Penny remembers her mother giving Penny's brothers "a lot of freedom." They fought with each other and other boys, shot BB guns at each other, used slingshots to zing apples at one another (one neighborhood boy nearly lost an eye). By the time they were teenagers, they drank and "caroused." She remembers her father as a "productive daily drinker," a carpenter who worked long hours earning money to support them all. The youngest, Penny felt like a tagalong, overshadowed, left out. She felt "fat, stupid, and ugly." She saw her brothers having fun. She wanted to be like them. "But I always got caught."

Doing what? I ask.

"Oh, throwing eggs at a teacher's house. Writing a nasty letter to my music teacher."

Penny is steeped in memories. She copes with her mother's failure of memory, but is also the literal keeper of "Mom's Memories," an audiotape she asked Mary to make years before, in the mid-1990s. Penny had been seeing a "professional listener"—her term for all psychotherapists. She'd just broken up with a boyfriend and was feeling depressed. As part of treatment, the therapist suggested good works. Penny saw an ad in the newspaper for hospice volunteers and remembers thinking, "I've got to do that. That'll be interesting." She even thought, "Maybe it will help me prepare for death," something Penny had long feared. ("My own, mostly, but I'm not too crazy about other people dying around me either.") She got trained and sat with dying people—she was babysitting, really—usually on Sundays while their families went to church.

She remembers one woman in the end stage of Alzheimer's. "She was a screamer," Penny says. "The family didn't warn me about that." A family member started a video on the TV, showed Penny the food she should feed the woman—"it was like oatmeal or something"—and left for church. From that moment, Penny says, the woman wailed, a rising tone that expended a whole breath, over and over.

The experience became salient for Penny, a memory that haunts her now as a caregiver, as she watches her mother's mind go. She remembers that the family of the wailing woman had built an addition on their house so that they could take her in. "I think of that now," she says to me. "I don't imagine [my mom] staying with me until the end—unless I had a whole lot more help. This whole staying-at-home thing is a really good idea." But she's not, she says, ever going to quit her job. Penny lives with an increasingly addled mother and tries to imagine the future, and the memory of the screaming woman turns wondering into worry and worst-case scenarios.

Volunteering for hospice gave Penny new appreciation for life's transience. She found herself anticipating losing her parents—and wanting a record of the past. She asked John and Mary to record their memories. Just tell stories, she pleaded. Her father refused— "he thought it was baloney"—but Mary sat at home and spoke into an old recorder. Penny lent me the tape. On it, Mary talks as a symphony plays on a radio in the background and a distant dog barks. Mary paints small scenes of her childhood, impressions of her mother, of losing her mother to cancer when Mary was four, growing up the youngest in a big Polish family, their father raising them alone, of running around with neighborhood kids, struggling through the Depression and the war, and of meeting Penny's father.

Near the middle of the tape is Penny's favorite moment. Mary recounts a story that took place before Penny was born, but which resonates deeply with Penny, the youngest child. She first listened to the story while driving from Connecticut to Wisconsin, returning from a visit to her parents. In it Mary talks about the birth of Deborah, the second child. Sophie, the oldest, was one. With the arrival of this small stranger in the house, Mary said, Sophie wouldn't eat:

After two days I called the doctor because Sophie didn't even go to the bathroom. This had me so worried. The doctor asked if we were doing anything different because of the new baby. We realized we had stopped playing the half hour or so before Sophie went to bed. So that night we took Sophie into the hide-a-bed with us and [played with her] and watched TV for a little. Then we put her to bed.

Well, the next morning I set before Sophie a soft-boiled egg and toast. She ate it. The tears rolled down my face.

Mary takes a breath and continues, in the low, warm voice that Penny knows so well, *So we knew what to do. That taught me a lesson. Every time I had another baby, my heart grew bigger. I loved all of you so much more. But I didn't know how to tell you that. I knew I grew bigger to hold the love, but I never could explain it to you.*

Listening in the car, Penny heard her mother speak of love expanding and cried.

On winter weekdays, this February of 2010, Penny arrives home from work in the late-afternoon dark. Pulling into the driveway, she spies her mother through the front picture window, Mary's face lit by the one water-pump lamp and the television set. Penny finds the sight of her mother's familiar head—its white hair, its particular shape and carriage—comforting. Penny is not yet an orphan, even if her mother is fading. Penny peers at the same head she's known for forty-nine and a half years. "I know someday I'm going to be grateful she was there," she says—meaning in Penny's home.

"Hell-o, Mommy!" Penny calls, opening the door.

"Hell-o," Mary says. Mary and Penny have similar voices, a bit gravelly, both nasal and melodic (a good voice for irreverent, funny stories).

In the kitchen, Penny deduces what her mother ate for lunch from the leavings: a banana peel, an empty pudding cup, dirty dishes. Penny cooks Mary dinner. She always cooks a protein and a vegetable, she says. They eat while watching the early news. Penny leaves the house again and drives to a six o'clock AA meeting. Meetings are her "savior," she says. So, too, she believes, was coming home.

"I could be dead by now," she reports during one of our almost-weekly lunches.

"If you hadn't come back?" I ask.

"Mm-hm. Easily. Yeah." This year she's "working the program" with more diligence. Increasingly she views taking care of her mother as a big part of the work. She's helping others, or at least *one* other. An important goal of the Twelve Steps, altruism doesn't come easy. Like recovery from addiction, it is One Day at a Time.

Back home, Penny watches TV with her mother.

Mary often asks—particularly with reruns on the Hallmark Channel—"Have you seen this?"

"Yeah, Ma," Penny often replies.

"Well, how could you see it without me seeing it?"

The familiar routine. "Mom, you *have* seen it."

"Well, I don't remember," Mary says matter-of-factly. She adds, "I can't remember shit."

CRS. Penny has heard the term thrown around in her plain-spoken family for longer than she can, well, remember. Before her mother's diagnosis, the term meant, simply, getting older: *Can't find my glasses. What's that actor's name?* Now CRS—can't remember shit—has become another way of talking about the vascular dementia—cognitive impairment from recurring, tiny strokes—that Mary has been diagnosed with. As the winter months pass, Mary asks more often, "Why can't I remember?" Over and over Penny hears the phrase, more plaintive than in earlier months.

"Because you have CRS," Penny says.

"Oh, that's right," Mary says. In her caregivers support group, Penny often calls her mother a "little Buddha."

Penny later confesses, "I can't tell if by 'Oh, that's right' she really understands. She knows what the expected response is."

Occasionally after an exchange like this, Mary grumbles, "You're just going to have to *put me down*."

"That used to really bother me, early on," Penny says. "I'd say, 'Mom, don't say that.'" Penny pauses, looking, as is her habit, for a reason to smile. "Then I started saying, 'Mom, it's not legal in this state. If we lived in Oregon, we might be able to swing something. But I'd have to pay off a few people. Because you're not that bad yet.'

"We do keep laughing. That's what my family does."

Penny walks through the living room. "What's going on now?" she asks her mother, pointing to the TV show.

"Ooh, I don't know; I can't follow it." Mary stares at the screen.

All the year and a half they've lived in this new house, Penny has *hated* the TV, the "mind-rot box," as she calls it. The sound of it, its pervasiveness, reminds her not just of how her life revolves around Mary, but of what Penny is losing: her mother, the living woman her mother used to be.

Every night before bed, Mary rolls her walker into the bathroom and brushes her teeth. Penny calls down the hall and reminds her mother to take her bedtime pills. Penny knows that Mary stands over the pill organizer, which Penny fills at the beginning of each week and leaves on the table next to the sink. Mary looks at the rows of subcompartments, marked with the days of the week. "She calls to me," Penny says, imitating her mother's voice, which means intensifying her own, "'*Is today Wednesday? Is today Thurs-*

day? Just *checking.'* I used to get annoyed. I want to say, 'Look it up on the calendar!' Then I'd think, 'Just answer her. Think what it's like to be in Haiti right now.'"

The month before, the devastating earthquake had killed more than two hundred thousand Haitians and left millions without food, housing, clean water. But knowing the intensity of others' suffering doesn't always lighten one's own—although it might help with one's response. Penny's mother is diminishing; Penny is a daily witness. She's trying to manage her mother's care—and bear long, slow loss—with skill and goodwill. She often wonders how much more she can take. What will tip the scales? Incontinence? She's already dealing with that. A fall? Her mother starting a fire in the kitchen? Penny figures at some point she'll need to move Mary to a facility. She just wishes she knew when the right time will be, and what is coming.

The uncertainty is hard, the going unpredictable. Penny will slowly find that in caring for another she herself becomes more steady and kind.

🌿 The Caregivers

Penny finishes work each day at four; her weekly caregivers support-group meeting begins at four. So she always arrives at the meeting a few minutes late. Every Thursday this winter she strides through the bright hospital lobby, past elevators, and down a hall where staff have hung landscapes by local artists. She turns right at a MAMMOGRAM AND BONE DENSITY sign, left at another set of elevators, and heads down another hall. The corridor is narrower here, the ceiling lower. The exposed pipes over Penny's head have been painted black, and the walls are, appropriately, hospital green. She passes food-prep staff working in small, fluorescent-lit offices. The air smells like fryers and sour grills. Across from a small cafeteria, she enters a bland, windowless conference room.

This is the hub of a wheel. In coming months, beginning in this room, friendships will forge, relationships will intertwine. In this subterranean space—shawl cold in summer, whirring and gusty with blowing heat in winter—sealed off from the world, women and men will tell private stories, offer weekly chapters in long sagas about their great daily burdens, interspersed by drama and death. Long-termers come weekly; others drop in every few months. Occasionally a visitor stops by, hears others' troubles, and never returns. I come along and stay for time enough that I almost feel I belong.

Benjamin Cooper, the group's moderator, usually bounces in five minutes late, just freed from a previous meeting. A compact man, balding, bearded, forty-five, he has an expressive, slightly elfish face. He has clipped his hospital badge—an I GOT MY FLU SHOT sticker on it—to his shirt pocket. An art therapist and the father of two school-aged children, he is the lead counselor in the "behavioral health unit" of the hospital, four floors above. Four years earlier, Ben had volunteered to moderate this group. He figured, presciently, that taking on new tasks would enhance his job security. Layoffs loom.

In the beginning, running the group, he was the "nervous support group leader." He knew nothing about caregiving, nor dementia and other diseases. Had someone asked, he wouldn't have been able to list, say, what every dementia caregiver should know about the progression of his or her charge's disease, or the risks that stress poses to caregivers' health. But he knew group dynamics, how to facilitate gatherings of strangers—the rest he learned on the job. By now his nervousness is gone. In meetings he listens, nodding. He offers advice rarely, asks questions occasionally, and more frequently offers short, affirming remarks. The comments often show

how well he knows the regulars. He'll refer in passing to Daniel's scholarship, William's wood carving, Inga's travels. "A lot of these people want to reclaim their lives," Ben says. Part of his job, he believes, is "learning who they were before." In months to come, he'll speak of feeling caught up in the members' lives. He'll attend funerals, visit caregivers and care recipients in hospital rooms, receive phone calls from group members during his busy workday. He'll worry occasionally that he's getting too involved, crossing professional boundaries. He is a facilitator, he reminds himself, not a therapist or a friend.

During this winter of 2010, a half dozen regulars typically sit around the table: Daniel, almost always at the end by the door closest to the way in; William, usually along the side nearest to the hall; Liz, often across from William; Ben frequently sits next to Daniel. Inga often ends up a few seats from Liz. Rufus usually strides in a little late and takes a seat by Liz and Inga. As the year progresses, ever more caregivers will join and stay. But at this point in the group's history, no more than eight people ever show up. The regulars, the caregivers—Penny, Daniel, William, Liz, Inga, and Rufus—fill the room with their stories.

🌿 Daniel

At her first support-group meeting, back in early 2009, Penny listened to eighty-eight-year-old Daniel "tell his life story." He became Penny's "most favorite guy. That's why I wanted to go back, just to hear him talk again." A retired professor of German, Daniel amazes the group with tales about his past. Members admire his stamina, his old-fashioned grace, and his intelligence—undiminished by age. He often arrives at the group earlier than the others and nods and tips his tweed cap toward each person who enters next: "Hi, Liz. How are you?" he says in a voice at once raspy, gentle, and somber. "Hello, Penny. Nice to see you." The group's love for him is magnified by their sense that he may not live much longer. "I don't know what kind of shelf life he has," Penny says in her matter-of-fact way. "He has some kind of slow-moving cancer."

He has non-Hodgkin's lymphoma and has lived with it for a decade.

He is thin and stooped, his skin translucent. He always wears slightly tattered corduroy pants, a button-down cotton shirt, a leather bomber jacket, and the tweed cap. His corduroys, while the correct length, fit wide on his skinny frame. He cinches his belt tight. His pants hang, the fabric bunching at the belt and draping over the scaffold of his hips. Daniel appears at first completely bald, but one day I notice fine hair growing around the back of his head, just above his nape. Liver spots fleck the rest of his smooth dome. Crust sometimes forms on his ears. The skin on Daniel's thin face closely traces the shape of his skull and is taut across his aquiline nose.

Daniel's large, bony, and elegant hands have long fingers. Nearly a century ago, his German father toured internationally as a piano accompanist for violinists and singers. His mother sang professionally, mostly German lieder. Daniel studied piano under his father's stern eye. He played a Haydn symphony, arranged for four hands, sitting with his father at the keyboard. Over and over, in a particular passage, Daniel got the rhythm wrong. *"Falsch! Falsch!"* his father cried, and Daniel tried again. His hands grew accomplished, intelligent.

When he speaks to the support group, he lifts his long fingers articulately. They hover over the table. One day this winter, he tells everyone that he's not doing well. "My wife is in the hospital," he says.

Daniel's caregiving has a twist. His wife, Leanne, is twenty-five years younger than he, in her early sixties. She is bipolar. She has other neurological problems, not definitively diagnosed, and still other health difficulties she has asked Daniel not to share with the group. She's in near-constant physical pain. She takes many medications. Figuring out the right ones, keeping track of them, managing the side effects—all of this is an enormous strain for Leanne, challenging for her doctors, and burdensome for Daniel, as are her fluctuating moods.

"She was severely depressed," he tells the group. "She said, 'Take me to the hospital.'"

He had driven Leanne along a winding road to a small hospital forty minutes away. The doctors checked her into a geriatric psychiatric unit—"a decent place," Daniel tells the group. He'd driven home alone.

"She has all kinds of physical ailments." He leans over the table and utters a version of a refrain he repeats nearly every week: "It's hard for me to take care of her—because I'm so old."

In the demographics of caregiving, Daniel is an outlier. The previous year, the National Alliance for Caregiving surveyed caregivers for people over fifty and found that only 5 percent were older than seventy-four. In his support group, however, Daniel's not demographically alone—although he is the oldest. Eighty-three-year-old William's wife is in a nursing home. Two other octogenarians will become regular members later in the year. The very old who care for the old cope with their own declining vitality—even serious health problems—*and* the needs of those who depend on them.

This winter of 2010, Daniel struggles with the everyday burdens of Leanne's mood swings, hospitalizations, and falls—and with housework and meal preparation, to which Leanne can barely contribute. He comes to the group each week and talks about his trials. He finds escape in his remarkable memories of prior decades, and comfort in music: he sits at home and listens to classical programs on public radio and selects favorite pieces from his shelves of CDs.

His caregiving will last only another year.

Daniel met Leanne when she was his graduate student in a summer tutorial. They married about two years later, in 1975. She had told him that she was manic-depressive (as bipolar disorder was called at the time). He says he didn't think much about it; she seemed fine. He remembers learning later that Leanne's first psychiatrist had told her that her illness would likely worsen as she got older. This turned out to be true. Other health problems came along as she aged. Daniel doesn't remember exactly how or when his role changed from husband to caregiver-husband. But one day in the late summer of 2008, after Leanne had become truly dependent on him, he noticed an ad for the support group in the local newspaper. In early meetings, often only he and two other men showed up. The men used to sit and talk about World War II. Eventually, toward the end of the hour, Ben recalls, the three would get around to discussing caregiving.

One of the other men was William. His wife, Joan, has Alzheimer's. A few years ago, Joan stayed for months in Ben's behavioral health unit. (The spouses of several other group members, including Daniel's wife, have spent time there, too. When group members refer to the place, they point to the ceiling and say "up there," as if indicating heaven, which of course it is not.) Later Joan moved to a nursing home. William visits her daily. He's a model in the group for his commitment to his wife, and also for finding enjoyment where he can. A retired builder, he makes wooden toys and birdhouses in his shop. For many years he has gotten together weekly with friends at a pizza place, where they play the state lottery, share a pizza, tell funny stories, and drink beer.

Daniel sees William's caregiving experiences—and those of the others whose spouses or parents have dementia—as very different from his own. Leanne's thinking is unimpaired. In this and other ways—background, education—he and William diverge. Still, Daniel finds solace in the group—in part, to his surprise, *because* of such differences. He's amazed by the gathering, sees it as uniquely American, "in the best way." A diverse bunch—male and female, financially secure and less so, gay and straight, liberal and conservative (although all white)—they come together as strangers and, through the weekly sharing of stories, develop not just relationships of support but, in many cases, friendships. Daniel believes such democratic openness would not have happened in Germany.

These days, with the group larger than it was when he joined, Daniel sits, listening to others' dilemmas, engaged but rarely commenting, his blue eyes staring at the table. He'll tell me later that as he sits and listens, he often plans just what he'll say.

William

"Today," William tells the group at one winter meeting, "Joan was trying to say, 'What are we doing here?' But it came out all wrong." He shakes his head, smiling. "I was trying to figure it out." Another day recently, he says, trying to clear clutter from the house, he discovered a handful of silver dollars in a little purse, and rolls of nickels, tucked away in the back of one of Joan's dresser drawers. Perhaps she'd squirreled them there, a symptom of her progressive disease, before she went to the nursing home.

Sixty-four years earlier, 1946: A friend of William's played in the Jimmy Perkins square-dance band. Jimmy called the steps. William's friend played banjo for some numbers, piano for others. William had been following the band around on weekend nights for six months, after he'd been discharged from the navy. One night he took a date to a dance in a small farming town north of his own. That night he also met Joan. "I fancied Joan, and the other girl fancied someone else—and that was it," he says. He remembers offering Joan a ride home. No, thanks, she said. Her father was coming to pick up her and her sister. William drove home. Later he heard that Joan and her sister had walked in the dark down Main Street. A car full of young men slowed alongside them. Joan and her sister hurried to a near house's front door and knocked. A woman let them in, and they called home for a ride.

William said to Joan later, "See? *I* would have brought you home."

He says, "We started going steady." This was, of course, a very long time ago. He tries to explain his attraction to Joan, and he's typically low-key and upbeat at the same time, as if by now it seems like mere common sense—something you've known for so long you don't know how you know it. "She seemed to be compatible with me. She had nice, long black hair. Real pretty. And those blue eyes. Yeah, she was good-looking. But she liked to do the same things I did, too."

William had served in the navy for two wartime years, stationed in Oakland, California, working supply. During his service, the right side of his face became paralyzed, and he spent six months in the hospital. "They couldn't figure out what was wrong with me. I couldn't close my eye at all. They sutured it together. They just made a little hole for me to see out of. And then it got a lot better." He shakes his head and smiles asymmetrically. "I have a crooked smile." He has a handsome face, calm, with gentle blue eyes. He's trim and looks much younger than eighty-three, wears jeans and neat, button-down shirts with the cuffs folded twice, to just above his wrists. One night during the war, in San Francisco with his navy buddies, he got a tattoo. Old and indistinct, it's just the vague shape of an anchor now. Sometimes it shows a little below the edge of his rolled right sleeve.

William married Joan in 1948. Soon William and Joan's father, a builder, constructed a house. William lives there still, sixty-two years later. Joan had, too, before she went to the nursing home. It's a small, white cape on an acre and a half, perched by a rural road. William became a contractor, too, and over five decades his company built more than a hundred homes around town. Driving on errands, he points out houses he built. He and Joan never had children. "We weren't that fortunate," he says, chuckling and shaking his head, as he often does when uttering sad words.

Wherever he goes, William carries two photographs of Joan and himself together. In his wallet, he keeps tucked a black-and-white picture from their wedding day, Joan in a white dress, a veil falling down her back, her dark eyebrows arcing. A heart-shaped face. The edges of the picture have frayed. The other photo appears whenever William opens his cell phone, which he draws from a holster on his hip. In it, Joan sits in her wheelchair at the nursing home, wearing a pink baseball cap and a pink sweatshirt. Her chin lifted, she looks at the camera. William leans in over her shoulder and smiles.

In September of 2006, William and Joan were staying at their vacation cottage on Cape Cod. William had been making repairs outside on the deck, and as he remembers it, the day skewed from the beginning.

Every time he walked into the house, he found Joan wandering around.

"I'm ready to go home," she said.

"It's not time to go home yet," William said. He went back outside.

For several years Joan had been increasingly muddled, withdrawn. During one of their annual trips to Florida in the motor home—journeys on which she always took sewing projects—she put down her needle and stopped quilting for good. Looking back, William figures she couldn't remember how.

Back then she and William were joining their friends every week at the pizza place, picking lottery numbers, and watching a TV screen to see if their choices came up. Joan always played the column of double digits that ended in seven. One day she couldn't remember and mulled over numbers that *began* in seven, too. It was the sort of quietly troubling incident that William noticed and simply coped with. Joan's primary-care physician had said something about Alzheimer's, but Joan had never been formally tested. She increasingly distrusted doctors. The last time Joan saw a doctor while she was still living at home, the physician had removed a growth from Joan's face. Leaving the clinic, Joan said to William, "I'm going to kill that woman." After that, William says, "you couldn't get her to a doctor, no matter what." William simply carried on, even after Joan was clearly losing herself. He took on more and more of the household tasks. Life was still manageable.

The day on Cape Cod, however, continued eerily. William worked on the house. He spied the cat, whom William usually kept indoors, down in the bushes near the car. "I had a job getting that cat back in," he says. Several more times, he had to capture the cat and deposit her back in the house. Inside, Joan was still distracted and confused. William told her he was going upstairs. He kept his ears tuned to the floor below. After a while, the house became strangely quiet—no sounds of activity, even from the dog. William hurried down and found the house unoccupied. He looked out the kitchen window. The cat was outside again, and the dog, too, and Joan stood in the sandy lot where William had parked the car.

He walked down the outside steps. "What are you doing?" he asked.

"I'm going home."

"How're you going to get there?"

"I'm going to take the car." But she was just standing there and had left the car keys in the house.

William sighed. "Okay. We'll go home. I'll get us ready." He started unwinding floats off the railing of the deck and tucking them under benches for the winter.

For some reason, William says, he sensed trouble. "I'm thinking, 'I've got to go in and see what's going on.'"

Joan was lurking in the kitchen. The headset of the corded wall phone was lying, off the hook, by the sink.

"What're you doing?" William asked, looking from Joan to the phone.

"I'm talking to the lady."

William picked up the phone. A 911 dispatcher was still on the line.

Joan started screaming from the other side of the kitchen, "He's got a gun! He's going to kill me!"

William was startled. He clutched the phone and said into it, "I don't have a gun. All my guns are at home." Joan kept yelling. "The operator could hear Joan, of course," William says.

"She's making a lot of noise," he said to the dispatcher.

"We'll send the police down," she said.

William hung up and told Joan that help was coming. She quieted. After what seemed to William a terribly long time, a police cruiser and ambulance trundled up the remote, beachfront road. A female EMT escorted Joan to the ambulance and talked to her inside it for twenty minutes or so. Two young male cops chatted with William up on the deck. "I don't have any guns down here," he assured them.

"They were nice," William says of the officers. "They said, 'We'll take her down to the hospital. You stay here for about thirty minutes, then you come down, too.'" William called one of Joan's sisters, who lived due west, across Cape Cod Bay. The sister drove southeast and William southwest, and they converged at the hospital. They waited with Joan for several hours in the emergency department. William said to a nurse, "If the doctors don't come soon, she's going to make a scene. It's not going to be pretty." A doctor did come soon. He asked questions that Joan couldn't answer. William remembers the doctor saying, "She's all right. Except she's got Alzheimer's pretty bad."

Back home, more trouble came. At first Joan's days were quiet again, although "one minute she'd know you, then the next minute she wouldn't," William says. "She'd go upstairs to bed and then come back down and say, 'When are you going home?' I'd say, 'Oh, I live here.'"

Not long after, William took their old, sick dog, Brittany, to the veterinarian, who put the dog down. "That was a bad day for Joan," William says. She had loved their many animals—a succession of springer spaniels and mutts, cats and parakeets, that she and William had nurtured, talked to, and traveled with over the years: Cuddles, Buffy, Sandy, Peanuts, Pepper, Tina, Chippy, Frisky, and others.

After they put Brittany to sleep, Joan went missing. William found her a half mile up the road, walking back from the house of a sister, who had already gone to a nursing home. Back in the house with the door locked, Joan threw a teakettle across the kitchen, and the cat dish and its contents onto the floor. In the dining room she pounded on a window, hard.

"That was scary," William says.

. . .

Joan was having a "catastrophic reaction." Sometimes dementia patients lash out, cry, go stubborn, or otherwise behave in extreme ways, in apparently ordinary situations. (Their alarm may also be expressed in milder ways.) The reactions come especially when a person is in or entering the middle stages of dementia—when she has both significant trouble functioning *and* enough awareness to be disturbed by this lack of functioning. As the brain loses ability, a person with dementia has ever lower "stress thresholds"—her calm becomes more and more fragile. Situations that once were navigable overwhelm her.

In the midst of Joan's outbursts that day, the phone rang, a welcome interruption. It was Joan's youngest sister, visiting a craft show in the area. She drove over, saw what was happening, and took Joan to the hospital. William stayed home and called a phone number he'd gotten from an area agency on aging, for a mental-health service. The social worker on the line asked William to meet her at the hospital. William drove over and answered her questions about what had been going on.

"By the time I got through with the interview, Joan was fine," William says. "But it was too late." Joan had been admitted to Ben's psychiatric unit on the fifth floor—"up there," as the group calls it—where she lashed out again. Doctors sedated her. William went home. In the next disturbing days, "she went downhill fast," William says. At first Joan "did a lot of crazy things" at the hospital, then she spent a lot of time sedated—not just calm, but out of it. She quickly lost her ability to walk, perhaps because of the medication. William is not sure. But once she had been sedated, Joan never walked again.

Alzheimer's patients who are hospitalized, as Joan was, are much more likely to decline, even die, quickly thereafter. Dementia patients need familiarity, predictability. Hospitals are confusing. During Joan's stay, a doctor at the hospital—William thinks that the physician was a general practitioner—predicted Joan would live only another six months or so. But more than three years later, Joan has proven him wrong.

At first William feared the psychiatric ward (he doesn't call it a loony bin, but that's his gist), but soon saw that the other patients—mostly young and committed to the ward because they'd been deemed dangerous to themselves or others—treated Joan kindly. "They liked her," he says. He felt grateful for this, but the place wasn't designed for dementia patients. He saw clearly, too, that he couldn't bring Joan home again. The doorways he'd built in his house were too narrow for a wheelchair, and he'd installed their one bathroom on the second floor. He felt he couldn't manage the catastrophes.

William had trouble finding a nursing home willing to take on Joan's agitation. She stayed in the hospital more than three months. On the day before their hospital-stay insurance would run out, a nursing home offered Joan a bed. William had had to learn fast how to afford a place: helped by an elder-care lawyer, he'd mastered the paperwork and "made poor Joan very poor," he says, so that she would qualify for Medicaid.

When Joan first moved to the nursing home, her teeth had long troubled her. She had nearly stopped eating and had slipped under a hundred pounds. William assented to the removal of all of Joan's teeth. With the teeth out, she started eating again. Her health stabilized, her behavior settled, and eventually doctors cut back her meds to nearly nothing.

"William kept Joan alive," his friend Claudia says. I have joined her, William, and her husband, Roger, one evening at their weekly gathering. "He really did. Because he went there every day. He reached out to her, made her eat."

William smiles, listening. "One of the girls"—he means an

aide at the nursing home—"says, 'I'm going to give you a badge that says you're a worker here.'"

He's one of the devoted ones.

❧ Liz

Liz admires William's devotion and herself attends the support-group meetings regularly, a committed member. But in coming months, for an important reason, she will feel she doesn't quite belong. She listens to spouses speak of love, longing, and grief over their loved ones' fates. Liz has her own difficult emotions, but they seem less acceptable to her, less easily shared. Only after many months will she fully disclose the reason she feels uneasy.

Her husband, Joe, moved to a veterans home the previous fall. This winter, she talks in the group meetings about Joe's trouble adjusting to the change, and her coping with unhelpful friends who have questioned her decision to move him. Liz has been coming to the group for about a year. Back then, weary and stressed, she had first dropped in on a monthly group specifically for Alzheimer's caregivers. But the people there talked about spouses who were already institutionalized, whose dementia was much further along. Liz didn't hear much that helped. At this weekly group, she found Daniel, Penny, Inga—people caring for family members with various illnesses, at varied stages. The meetings focused on the general challenges of giving care, which she preferred.

She and Joe met through friends in the late 1980s or early '90s—Liz can't remember exactly. She'd been living alone in her small ranch home a few miles from downtown. Her first husband had died a decade earlier. Her three children were grown. Joe was a contractor—a "master carpenter," Liz says. Over the next few years he did small projects for her around the house. A year would pass and Liz wouldn't see him. Then in 1994 she noticed her crumbling roof. She called Joe. "Any chance I can get you to fix it?" she remembers asking. Sure, he said.

Climbing down from the roof one day, he asked, "How'd you like to go out sometime?"

Liz recalls feeling taken aback. It had been years since she had even been on a date. She had settled into a self-sufficiency that felt secure.

Plus, you're my *handyman,* she thought. "Can I get back to you on that?" she asked.

"Okay."

She called him a few days later. "I'll go out with you," she remembers saying. "But I can't make you any promises, okay?"

"Okay," he said.

Two years later, they married on Saint Lucia in the Caribbean, at a fancy resort on the beach. Joe had been married before, too. It was, for each of them, their first trip to the Caribbean, and it gave them "a bug for the islands," Liz says. For the next five years or so, they traveled several times a year.

But meanwhile Liz's chronic pain had begun. Four months after the wedding, she got a severe headache, and it persisted for days. She saw a doctor. Pain relievers helped but not completely. She checked into the hospital. "Nobody could figure out what it was. They said, 'We'll treat it as a full-blown migraine.' But it never went away."

It didn't. "I've had a headache for fourteen years," Liz says. Soon her body began reacting to the medications she had been prescribed. Her options for managing the pain diminished. She applied and qualified for disability benefits. She quit her job as a medical assistant.

This winter the pain gets so bad sometimes that she stays in bed all day. Most of the time, she perseveres through errands and housework, tolerating the dull ache around her forehead and temples. "I remember saying to Joe, 'My headaches will get better, and then you'll get something.' But I was *kidding*."

She first noticed Joe's forgetfulness during a vacation in the Caribbean.

"Time to get ready for dinner, Joe," she said one evening.

"Right." Ten minutes later he was still sitting in their hotel room.

"Joe, I said it's time to get ready for dinner. Don't you remember me saying it before?"

"No."

During one meal on that trip, he and Liz chatted with a couple they'd met; they talked about Canada, where the couple lived. A few moments after the conversation had turned to another topic, Joe asked, "So where are you two from?"

Back home, he got out fertilizer from their garden shed. Liz said, "It's supposed to rain in a couple of days. Why don't you wait until then to use it?"

"Sure."

He fertilized anyway.

"What are you doing?" Liz asked.

"I'm putting the fertilizer on!"

"We just talked about that!"

But Joe had forgotten.

"He'd get mad," Liz says. She would, too.

She made an appointment with Joe's doctor, who sent Joe to a neuropsychologist. Joe took fourteen tests for memory and cognition. On the tests, he had some difficulty learning new information and retrieving it later. He told the neuropsychologist that he often felt anxious, sometimes panicky, getting his job done. He was working as a locksmith at the time. Overall the clinician found nothing major wrong. In his report, he wrote that the exam results suggested "mild cognitive impairment, potentially indicating the early stages of a progressive process."

This was in 2003. Joe was sixty-seven. Two years later, with Joe's confusion worse, Liz brought him to a neurologist, who ordered a brain scan. The doctor wanted to rule out a mass or a blood clot. The scan was fine, Liz says. She remembers that the neurologist said, "I go more by what the family tells me." He also tested Joe's memory. Liz remembers he asked Joe to spell the word *world* backward—part of the standard "mini mental-status exam" used to identify dementia. Joe wasn't able to. The neurologist diagnosed Alzheimer's.

Inga

Inga is a caregiving veteran. One day she introduces herself to a support-group newcomer, an elderly woman whose husband has had a stroke. "So as not to confuse you," Inga says, "I'll try to be clearer than I have been before with others." Inga is seventy, has long, thick silver hair and startlingly blue eyes. She pauses and leans slightly across the table toward the new woman. "I'm gay."

"You're what?"

"I'm *gay*. I'm a lesbian."

"Oh!" the newcomer says cheerfully. "So what? I'm straight." She chuckles. Everyone laughs.

Inga says, "Well, before, when I've talked about [my partner] Louise, people asked me, 'Is she your *daughter*? Is she your mother? Is she your granddaughter?'"

"Everything but," the woman says.

"Everything but." Inga gives an emphatic nod. "Okay," she says, as if glad the facts have been established. "I've been a caregiver for my *partner*, Louise, for about ten years. I was at rock bottom two years ago. These people saw me at my worst in November of 2008."

Rufus and Ben nod.

"My partner has had atrial fibrillation, heart ablation, pacemaker, breast cancer, skin cancer, left-hip replacement, left-hip replacement removal, cement spacer, left-hip replacement redo, right-hip replacement." Inga pauses. "That's about it. Over the ten years."

"In addition to MRSA," Rufus says, "and adverse drug reactions."

Ben adds, "And a little depression."

"A lot of depression," Inga says. "So anyway, she nearly died. At this time, she is almost well. She's able to walk. She is able to take care of her personal affairs." Inga smiles. "And we're getting married!"

"Oh, how nice," the newcomer says, smiling.

"We're celebrating her being alive and we're celebrating thirty years together by getting married." It's Massachusetts in 2010, after all—six years after the state became the first to legalize gay marriage.

"That," Inga says, "is my story."

MRSA stands for methicillin-resistant *Staphylococcus aureus,* a strain of bacteria that lives on the surface of many people's skin without causing problems. Sometimes the bug causes serious infections, particularly in people with weaker immune systems and in hospitals and other medical settings. MRSA does not respond to most antibiotics, and many people who contract it do not recover. Some die; others live with the infection, kept at bay through surgery and other treatments, for many years.

Louise had gone into the hospital in 2008 for a hip replacement. After the surgery, she was transferred to a nursing home for physical therapy and rehabilitation. Louise did well in rehab and came home on schedule. But later Inga became concerned about the appearance of Louise's surgical site. Several weeks after the surgery Louise's wound broke open. Inga brought Louise to the surgeon's practice, where a physician's assistant examined her. He was unconcerned. Inga remembers him saying, "That's not an infection, really. It's like squeezing a pimple."

Inga described for the PA the extent of the discharge at home. "He said, 'Take Tylenol, monitor it, she'll be fine.'"

"I said, 'Please look at it under a microscope.'"

"He said, 'Come back in a week.'"

Inga and Louise left. No testing of the discharge happened.

A week later, the wound had not improved. Back at the surgeon's office, the PA was still untroubled. Later that day Inga and Louise stopped by the office of Louise's primary-care physician. He looked at the wound, took a sample to be cultured, and days later called Inga. "This is not good," she remembers him saying. "Louise has MRSA."

Months of treatment followed. During a first hospital stay, a surgeon removed Louise's hip joint. In the space created, he installed a cement block infused with antibiotics. "The head of infectious disease [at the hospital where Louise had the surgeries] took a personal interest in her case," Inga says. She credits this specialist's help with Louise's recovery. "On December thirty-first, 2008," Inga says, "Louise was declared MRSA-free. She had set something of a record, recovering from a MRSA-infected hip replacement." Louise's doctor had said that everybody he had ever treated with MRSA was either, as Inga puts it, "six feet under or in a wheelchair and getting recurrent infections."

In January of 2009, Louise and Inga "started all over," Inga says. A surgeon pulled out the cement block and installed in Louise a fabricated hip. Louise went back to a nursing home for rehab. She endured five more surgeries and five follow-up stays in nursing homes. Between each rehab and each subsequent surgery, she stayed at home, and Inga cared for her.

Meanwhile Inga was her partner's care manager and advocate. She updated friends and family, all of them distant, on Louise's progress and treatments. She kept the house clean and paid bills and dealt with insurance claims. The care consumed her days. Along the way Inga had read, in the local paper, a notice about a support group for caregivers. She admitted to herself that she needed to go. She was, she realized, "falling apart."

Dependence

On a Thursday during this February of 2010, Ben draws the shades on the windows of the doors to the conference room and takes his seat. It is a small group today; only William, Inga, Rufus, and Penny have shown up. When it is her turn, Penny announces, "My mom lost a tooth." She reaches into her jeans pocket and pulls out a plastic baggie. "I have it here, in fact. Anybody want to see it?"

The others don't leap at the chance, but Penny passes the baggie to her left. Rufus examines it.

"It's *most* of a tooth," Penny says.

She comes to these meetings, she tells me, because she likes sharing stories with people who understand. "You've got this miserable thing," she says—sort of like bereavement, but instead you're *anticipating* a final loss. "You're dealing with the inevitable. This is going to end in death." The people here know instinctively just to be present for others' experiences—their stories, complaints, and worries, no matter how apparently trivial: the tooth, the pill, the eternal cleaning up, the food, the lack of sleep.

Rufus holds up the small wedge of Mary's tooth, encased in plastic, between his fingers. "It snapped right off," he says. A Civil War reenactor, Rufus has a beard and a scraggly mustache, the whiskers falling just below his chin. They help him look authentic in his Union blues. He's a Republican among Democrats, can't stand Obama, quotes Shakespeare and Ogden Nash, talks about once working at the Veterans Administration, and rails against bureaucracies. He tells every newcomer that for seven years he cared for a friend, a fellow reenactor, with Lou Gehrig's disease. The friend died several months ago. Rufus keeps coming back.

"It doesn't bother her at all," Penny says of the missing tooth. "Do you think it's a canine?" She watches as the bag goes from Rufus to Inga, who inspects briefly and passes it on to William.

"I'm not going to go looking in her mouth to see!" Penny says.

A mouth is a private place. Perhaps the most basic dynamic of caregiving is dependence, one person on another. In elder caregiving, it is *new* dependence, the result of decline. Someone once independent becomes reliant on another. With dependence comes heightened, often unwanted, intimacy. Penny cares for her mother's body in ways similar to how Mary long ago cared for Penny—feeding, reminding, watching for signs of illness. But though so many of the basic acts are similar to mothering, the tone of elder caregiving is sorrow, not joy. Human beings—perhaps especially American human beings—don't like decline. We admire growth, the evolution from helplessness to independence. The child grows out of dependency, emerging from formlessness into what we think of as the true adult condition: identity, agency, an ability not just to take care of oneself, but to make things happen. We call this state dignity: possessing an independent, upright, physically capable self, worthy of respect.

The phrase *role reversal*, then, for describing a child's care for a parent, while useful, seems far too simple. It misses the parent's frequent desire for competence, her memory of her previous capacities, the parent's and the child's complicated emotions about their shifting duties—the role *messiness* that arises. Mothers, fathers, daughters, sons—each with their memories, histories, presumed jobs, and preferences—muddle through new roles.

Weeks after passing her mother's tooth around to the group, Penny will find out that the little shard was not a real tooth, but a prosthetic one that had broken off of Mary's partial-plate dentures. This surprises Penny: for all the heightened intimacy Penny now has with her mother—more intimacy than Penny wishes for—this detail had escaped her. It will, in retrospect, seem like something her mother should have been able to *tell* her—rather than something Penny would find out by poking around in Mary's mouth.

"At their outer reaches," writes Wendy Lustbader in *Counting on Kindness: The Dilemmas of Dependency,* "shame and intimacy converge." Daughters and sons may recoil from closeness with their parents' bodies, with those bodies' functions. Adult children may feel shame—shame on behalf of the parent, shame for oneself. They may resent that their lives are taken over by their parents' bodily needs. Until now the child's job had been to break out and establish his or her life. Now there is this coming back, this cleaning up, this watching over, being pulled away from one's "own" life. Ben will speak, in the coming months, about the value of professional care: it helps daughters preserve their roles as daughters, husbands their roles as husbands, and so on.

This may be a white, particularly middle-class, American ideal. Latino caregivers, for example, who make up 10 percent of American caregivers, seem to spend more time than whites do helping with messy activities such as bathing and toileting. Yet they also tend to see their care in more positive ways and take longer to move their family members to institutions than whites do. African-Americans (who make up 11 percent of US caregivers) report less stress and depression, and greater rewards, in caregiving than whites do. Many African-Americans report turning to their religious beliefs for solace; perhaps faith elevates the way they see their roles and burdens.

Not just Penny's race and ethnicity, but her particular family culture, shape her outlook, too. A raucous familial humor may make caring for her mother a little easier. Her siblings, she says, don't shy from sharing details about their bowel functions, for example—they're good fodder for laughs. The humor eases one aspect of caring for her mother, although it is still the most burdensome.

Penny first describes the "blowouts" to me during one of our weekly lunches. Not many people can chuckle over dealing with a parent's incontinence and munch salad at the same time, but Penny can and does. She recounts for me the worst episode yet: She had asked her mother to ride on an errand to a nursery. Penny needed to pick up plants she had ordered, and she wanted Mary to get out of the house. At first Mary resisted; she would just sit at home with the TV, thank you.

"Come on," Penny said. "It's a beautiful day."

So Mary sat in the car. Penny drove, parked, and went in to chat with the nursery's owner.

"We weren't there five minutes before she started blowing the horn," Penny says.

"I've got to *go!*" Mary said to Penny back at the car. Penny told the nursery owner she had to leave. He offered his bathroom.

Penny looked at the rickety, steep stairs leading to the bathroom. "No, thanks. My mom uses a walker. I think we'd better drive home."

In the car, Mary, sitting in the passenger seat, complained, "Oh, it's bad."

"Well, if you've got to let go, let go." Penny drove as fast as she dared. She pulled into her driveway and helped Mary out of the car. Mary started her slog up the steps. Penny stood behind her mom, reaching to hold open the storm door. "And then it's coming out," Penny says, "over her *shoe,* onto the *step*. It was like *lava*. It was like a *volcano*. Like, *rrraah*. Coming out."

She and Mary made their way into the house. Penny lowers her voice and gestures at an imaginary floor with her hand. "There were little plops, through the living room, through the kitchen, the hallway, into the bathroom." Seeing that Mary wasn't making it to the toilet in time, Penny had said, "Oh, my God. Oh, man."

Mary said, "I'm sorry."

Penny said, "Mom, don't be sorry. It's part of life. Shit happens."

Penny says to me, "It could have been worse. She could have hit the only carpet we have, when you come in the door. She could have hit the bath mat."

Penny spent hours cleaning. "Shoes, socks, washcloths, pants, underwear. I took it all downstairs. Dealt with it in the giant sink."

Things could *always* be worse, Penny thought. "I said, 'Mom, it was only one leg. It could have been down both legs of your pants. It happened at home,'" not at the nursery. "'What kind of friends would we have made with that guy if we'd stayed, huh, Mom?' We laughed about it for the rest of the day."

🌿 Of Care and Cure

Cleaning up after incontinence may be the most private and unspoken of caregiving tasks—a source of quiet shame. Certainly for Penny it is the greatest source of resentment. Her irritation is exacerbated by her isolation—from her siblings, her community— the feeling that she is going it alone, without direct support or even shared experience.

Likely throughout history, people have abhorred the tasks of cleaning up when the body is messy. But in earlier America, illness and care for the sick were more visible and communal affairs. Medicine was domestic and in the hands of women (men did care for the ill, but their involvement was an exception to a rule), and caregiving a central element of what historian Emily Abel calls "collective female life." Women followed an oral tradition of remedies and treatments, passed down through generations. They applied salves, cleaned wounds, brewed herbal tinctures, learned from one another—and took turns sitting with the dying.

In the nineteenth century, by the time women reached adulthood, they would likely have witnessed the deaths of as many as a hundred people and helped care for scores of these. Siblings, other family members, and neighbors often fell ill from infectious disease, and the very sick often died. In colonial America, one in eight women died in childbirth, and one in eight to ten children died before the age of five. Death and illness, while certainly causes for grief and anxiety, were more commonplace in early America, viewed as nearly normal. Fewer people lived to old age.

Not just *trends* in illness, deaths, and caregiving, but *attitudes* toward sickness and old age have shifted enormously, as well. As historian Thomas Cole writes in his Pulitzer-nominated book, *The Journey of Life: A Cultural History of Aging in America,* a basic dichotomy has governed American views of aging—with esteem of healthy and self-reliant old age at one end, and disdain for decay and dependence at the other. (The latter state, in earlier times, was associated with sin, and in more recent times, failure.) The basic dualism has endured, even as the frame has shifted from a spiritual to scientific one.

Puritans brought to the New World a belief that their destinies were determined by God. They had a "cosmological" view of the end of life and, as Cole writes, "urged early American believers to seek spiritual strength and personal growth by accepting frailty and decay as inevitable aspects of flawed human existence." Yet the Puritans also planted the seeds of self-reliance and individualism. Their view included the emerging belief that everyone journeys individually through life, seeking and earning salvation and thereby, in some sense, determining his or her fate.

With the Enlightenment came rationalist, scientific ideals, the concept of the "self-made man" independent of the circumstances of his birth—and hopes that science would conquer all disease. Cole cites Benjamin Franklin, who wrote of "the power of man over matter."

"All diseases," Franklin opined, "may by sure means be prevented or cured, not excepting even that of old age, and our lives lengthened at pleasure."

As Victorians "conquered" the West and developed industry and cities, they prized civilized morality, faith, and correct social behavior as guarantees of "a good old age and its religious rewards." Illness, in this context, equaled moral failing. Some of Cole's descriptions of Victorian attitudes remind me of my grandmother Hildegard. Her father, born in Germany in 1866, emigrated to Pennsylvania as a young man and, with a business partner, founded an entire town and textile industry. In late life he was a philanthropist. In some ways, he lived the Victorian ideal. He passed on to his offspring—my grandmother, and me—ideas about vitality, goodness, independence. Old age to Victorians, Cole writes, "represented an embarrassment to the new morality of self-control."

I also see my grandmother, and her decision to end her life, in Cole's descriptions of our current scientific era's attitudes toward old age, in which standards of "normal" or "successful" aging are set (in theory) by objective scientific research. The burgeoning of science and scientific medicine has reinforced the ideal espoused by Franklin: that we can beat any disease. There's the sense that we *should* stay young and well, as long as we consult the best doctors, take the right medicines, eat the correct foods, and possess upbeat attitudes. In this context, illness and dependency are framed as failures of either medicine or an individual's will. "Stated baldly," Cole writes, American attitudes toward aging have been a "historical evolution from communal ideals of transcendence through societal ideals of morality to individual ideals of health." Old age, Cole writes, has become a problem to be solved, as opposed to a mystery or existential condition to learn how to live with.

Meanwhile, from the eighteenth into the twenty-first century, the family caregiver's role radically changed. Until the late nineteenth and early twentieth centuries, medicine was not an organized profession. Doctors worked independently, were far-flung geographically, did not need to be licensed, and had eclectic approaches to healing, writes the sociologist Paul Starr in his seminal book *The Social Transformation of American Medicine: The Rise of a Sovereign Profession and the Making of a Vast Industry.* Americans, particularly rural Americans, generally had little access to physicians. Even when they did, they often resisted doctors' services, out of self-reliance and a distrust of practitioners who were unfamiliar. Households mostly relied on the skills and traditional knowledge of their own family and other community members.

Starr describes a shift that occurred in the nineteenth and into the twentieth centuries—and paralleled other social and economic changes. Medical knowledge, once seen as the domain of women caring for the ill at home, became the domain of a growing profession of physicians working under uniform standards and licensing requirements, within new institutions—hospitals. Care for the ill and aged occurred increasingly in a public, bureaucratized, market-driven sphere. "Sickness and insanity, childbirth and death," became segregated from everyday life, Starr writes. The creation of the medical profession and its industry was part of an overall "rationalization" of society, a removal of "disturbances" from domestic life, he argues, so that healthy people might participate fully in industrial society.

Along the way, family caregivers became accessories to professional medicine. Penny is thus responsible for her mother, yet authority concerning Mary's care lies elsewhere, in the public, expert, specialized sphere. Just as the home in general has become more isolated, the twenty-first-century caregiver now works at the social margins.

Not that Penny would want to return to the nineteenth century. She is, after all, a professional herself, earning a living through her expertise in a refined area. She, and surely most women, would reject the idea of returning to nineteenth-century caregiving, which bound women to the home perhaps more than any other domestic obligation. But today's arrangement brings with it particular burdens: caregivers' work is isolated, often lonely, and perhaps more psychologically taxing than it was for those nineteenth-century women living collective lives. In the nineteenth century, women moved in and out of one another's homes, shared information and resources, took turns relieving one another in caring for their children, and their ill and dying. In contrast, Penny alone shuttles Mary between home and the private, clinical rooms where Mary meets with specialists. Penny's communication with most of her distant siblings consists of occasional updates by e-mail. She drives to her job in another town and tries to—must—keep her paid work separate from her caregiving at home.

Shifts in attitudes toward informal care paralleled the changes in views on aging that Cole writes about. Nineteenth-century women did what they could for their loved ones and then, to a large extent, surrendered the rest to God, says Elizabeth Sharpe, a historian who has studied nineteenth-century women's written accounts of caregiving. Sharpe was struck by her subjects' relative lack of angst. Unlike contemporary caregivers, no woman in Sharpe's research described feeling conflicted about her obligation to her family member, or "clueless" about how to help. No one said she was afraid or felt guilty that she hadn't done enough. No one wrote of feeling *responsible for everything*, Sharpe says—for finding the right medicines, keeping her family member entertained, achieving the right diagnosis. The women's accounts, although they describe physical suffering and difficult work, express little psychological insecurity. The women may have disliked the work, even resented it—but they seem free of significant inner conflict about their roles or obligations. They were even, perhaps, empowered by the expertise they did possess. Meanwhile they were soothed by a more "cosmological" worldview and left their charges' fates in the hands of God.

In contrast, Penny and the other caregivers in her support group—particularly the women—often worry and feel guilty and insecure about the care they give. As health-care deputies rather than recognized medical experts, coping with feelings that caregiving competes with whatever else they *should* be doing, Penny and others may *try* not to complain. But in this context, acceptance comes hard.

Perhaps it was easier for women in those earlier, religious times because one's fate was presumed out of one's hands. Many Americans today are as religious as their nineteenth-century counterparts, but members of Penny's Massachusetts support group rarely mention faith, or God, as they cope with their circumstances. This is likely for a number of reasons: The setting of the support group is a secular hospital, not a church. The group represents a diversity of beliefs, which may inhibit any assertion of one's own. The members are a sample of their quite secular town and region. And finally, religious caregivers in the community may seek support first at their churches, synagogues, and temples, rather than heading to a hospital conference room.

Penny, not a churchgoer, does in her own, twenty-first-century way seek guidance from, and practice surrender to, a "higher power." She's led by one of AA's central prayers: "God, grant me the serenity to accept the things I cannot change, the courage to change the things I can, and the wisdom to know the difference." Acceptance, subordinating her ego to a greater force, is a big part of her recovery work, a central theme in AA. "I don't realize my life's not my own," she says—meaning, her life is largely not hers to control. "The only thing I have control over right now is my attitude. There's nothing I can do about how my mom progresses. I can just take it day in, day out, and do what I can."

At the same time, all the acceptance talk gets old. Friends in AA tell Penny, "You have to accept it"—your situation.

"I say, 'You have to accept that I have to whine every once in a while!'"

Aging, illness, and dependence happen, in defiance of science and American ideals. Dependence often lasts long. Illness in old age leads frequently to partial recovery, followed by a tenuous stability, another slide, another recovery, and so on, until eventually, after years of decline, illness leads to death. Along the way the word *cure*—as Suzanne Mintz, executive director of the National Family Caregivers Association, points out—becomes irrelevant.

The word's history parallels the history of medicine and caregiving. *Cure* originally meant "care and concern," particularly spiritual care. Only later did it come to signify "successful medical treatment," the *removal* of disease. What once meant "to take care of" came to mean "to fix." By necessity, despite medical advances, Penny and Mary are living the older meaning.

Before Penny had moved back in with her mom, people in Wisconsin had said, "It's so nice of you to go and spend your mother's last years with her." Penny had thought, My mother's last years? What do you mean? Not long after, living with Mary, Penny found herself in tears. Her mother had said something—Penny can't recall exactly what—that "didn't compute, something that she didn't remember, that I really thought she should." Penny pointed the lapse out to her mother, and Mary said, "Oh, I'm just *kidding*."

"Mom, no, you're not," Penny recalls saying. "The hard thing is, I'm watching you lose it, a little bit every day."

🌿 Refugee

Daniel says to the group at a winter meeting, "I have a severe case of sciatica," terrible pain in his lower back and leg. "Has any of you ever wrestled with this?"

"I have!" Rufus says.

"What did you do?" Daniel asks.

"Screamed and yelled!" Rufus also saw a physical therapist. "I did everything she told me to do," but it hardly helped. "Then, I was sleeping on a cot at camp"—this would be a reenactment camp—"and I woke up, and—I could stand up!" He was cured. Apparently, sleeping on a nineteenth-century cot adjusted his spine.

Rufus believes in this odd cure, but still says to Daniel, "You need a good physical therapist."

"Yeah. Okay," Daniel nods.

Liz says, "Dr. Connor. Riverside Sports and Physical Therapy. Main Street." Daniel takes a piece of paper from his wallet and carefully writes this information down.

• • •

After the meeting, I ask Daniel if I may walk out with him. He shuffles slowly, stepping and leaning on his cane. We pass the food-service offices. I ask if he's in pain right now.

"A bit, but it's not excruciating."

"Did you take anything?"

"Just some aspirin," he says. Another step. And another. Still new to the meetings, I forget which way to go at an intersection. "This way." We turn right. "It's confusing," he says to reassure me.

He recalls his years of teaching German at a university. He taught undergraduates mostly. "There's a language requirement, so the students are unmotivated. There's a lot of psychological resistance." He says languages should be taught at the elementary level, when students still aren't "inhibited."

We pass the hospital's main stairway. "You immigrated from Germany?" I ask.

Daniel stops walking for a brief moment, as if knowing that what he'll reply carries impact. "I was a refugee from Nazi Germany."

"Oh." I ask which year, because it matters.

"Nineteen thirty-four," he says. Very early in Hitler's reign.

"Did you escape with family?"

"My brother and I. My father came later. My mother had died years before." He takes a few steps. "We were very lucky."

We've walked all the way to radiology. Just ahead are chairs. He seems tired. "I don't want to keep you from resting," I say.

"Yes, I think I need to stop." He stands, stooped, before a chair, facing me.

I thank him for answering my questions. "I hope you feel better. I hope your wife feels better."

Daniel lifts a hand, takes the brim of his cap in his fingers, makes a little bow, and tips his hat just so. "Thank you." He smiles and lowers himself into the chair.

• • •

Through the winter, storms roll up the East Coast and into New England. Snow piles up along the town's streets and sidewalks. Ice threatens on front steps. It's a hard time to be old. This winter Daniel copes, too, with Leanne's falls. In the middle of one night, she slips in the bathroom. "The room is so small," Daniel says to everyone. "It was hard for me to figure out how to help her. I pushed that button"—a medical alert button. Leanne had fallen a month ago, too. An ambulance and several EMTs had arrived at the house. It had seemed to Daniel an unnecessary commotion. "This time they used their heads," he says. "They sent a policeman. He just picked her up and asked her to sign something that said she wasn't hurt. The next morning, she hardly remembered.

"She's overmedicated. She takes Ambien. She sleepwalks. If she doesn't go right to sleep after she takes the Ambien, she staggers." He draws a breath. "I can't pick her up. She can't pick herself up because her legs are too weak." He shakes his head slowly and smiles a close-lipped smile. "Marriage is a roller coaster. At least mine is. We pick ourselves up and go on from there, as if nothing had happened."

Early on in their marriage, he and Leanne had a lot to talk about with each other. Leanne's father had been an ordained pastor. Instead of leading a congregation, he ran the National Conference of Christians and Jews. Leanne and Daniel connected around ecumenical values and scholarship: Leanne used to help Daniel write his academic papers and books. "She was a taskmaster!" he says.

One year, while he was writing a book on Gustav Mahler, struggling to get it done, she said to him, "Go to the library every day. Work in your carrel for three hours a day. Keep a log of your work. It will get done."

He did what she said, and finished the book on time.

"She was right," he says.

In recent years, with Daniel retired, Leanne helped him organize lectures on the Holocaust. But "those talks are over now," Daniel tells the group. This is a problem because the work had motivated Leanne, given her a sense of worth, some aspiration. Among the most burdensome aspects of Daniel's caregiving is the fact that he is helping a woman survive who doesn't want to live. He reports that Leanne says occasionally, "Once you go, I'm not going to stick around."

It's a disquieting statement. The group just listens. "Suicide runs in her family," he says. Later in the winter, a doctor admits Leanne again for an inpatient psychiatric stay. A friend had driven Daniel and Leanne to a hospital in Cambridge for a consultation about other health problems. After meeting with Leanne, the physician asked to speak with Daniel. "Leanne was sitting there looking very unhappy," Daniel tells the group. "While we were talking, men came with a gurney." They wheeled Leanne away, still wearing her street clothes and holding her cane.

Ben, who has been hearing about Leanne's suicide talk for a couple of years now, says, "I'm very sorry to hear about that, but a little relieved, too."

"I think the doctor was completely justified," Daniel says. "She was in bad shape. The medications weren't right. I'm hoping that during this hospital stay they'll straighten them out."

Ben asks how Daniel's doing.

Daniel takes a breath. "I'm at loose ends. I sit and listen to music most of the time."

"You need to go play keno and drink some beers with William," Ben says, smiling at William. Ben often encourages group members to take time away from caregiving, to find ways to enjoy themselves.

William smiles. "It helps!"

Daniel looks over at William and nods.

Daniel's challenges surge and subside from day to day. Two weeks after he reports to the group that Leanne was hospitalized, he takes a deep breath and says, "Things are difficult. Leanne is back home." She lies on the couch, uncomfortable. Daniel glances at Ben. "She can be abrasive. But that's nothing new."

Ben nods. He asks if Leanne is still driving.

Daniel chuckles. "She drives to *McDonald's.*" She descends two steps to the garage, gets herself into the car, and motors to the drive-through. "She gets a *biscuit,*" he says, shaking his head, smiling.

It is a recurring theme for Daniel: food. It intersects with the labors of marriage, with emotions and power struggles. He sometimes apologizes to the group for talking about something so trivial. But after seventy-six years in America, he still doesn't like his adopted country's food, neither the fast food that Leanne craves, nor the gourmet dishes they find at the restaurants they go to occasionally. "I hope I won't offend anyone with this," he says one day. "But the food in this country is *drowned* in heavy sauces and creams. I can't eat it. I grew up on spare food: cabbage and potatoes. Leanne will put *ketchup* on her french fries." He shakes his head, as if this practice were outlandish.

The group laughs.

"I would never do that. Even the *sight* of it . . ." He waggles his head again. "She's welcome to eat it that way, but . . ." He pauses, thinking of another offense: The hospital coffee shop has "the best apple pie. And they have to put *ice cream* on it! I would never dream of it. It would ruin the ice cream *and* the pie."

Liz and Penny smile.

Six years ago, Daniel became a vegetarian, although he eats fish occasionally. I ask him one day why he decided to stop eating meat. He tucks his chin, thinks for a moment. "I think the best explanation is that I love animals. And I don't think they get treated well. I know that there is a movement afoot to change that, but I think it will take a long time."

To the group he says, "So Leanne said tonight she is going to make an omelet. I said, 'Okay, but nothing but an omelet.' She said, 'Well, let's make it a *mushroom* omelet.'"

Rufus leans forward and raises his eyebrows. "And?"

"I haven't gone home and eaten it yet." Daniel raises his eyebrows also and smiles his befuddled smile. "I'm supposed to buy the mushrooms."

The group laughs. In intimate relationships, even trivialities such as mushrooms can take on weight.

Daniel does what Liz suggested: he makes an appointment with Dr. Connor at Riverside Sports and Physical Therapy. Daniel receives a cortisone shot, which relieves his sciatica. The following week, he tells the group how grateful he is for the advice. He also describes his latest challenge: "We lost the most recent home health aide. She didn't show up, which usually means they're not going to come back. We were on good terms with her. She could have just picked up the phone and said, 'I can't come.' I left her a message in the morning."

She never showed up.

Penny recommends the elder-care agency she uses. Daniel

writes, but he has a hard time understanding the name Penny is pronouncing.

"Do you want me to write it down?" Daniel passes Penny his slip of paper, and she writes.

Later Daniel tells me that he finds it difficult to come up with solutions to day-to-day problems, even to follow through on solutions the group suggests. "I'm not very practical." But he seems to find comfort in simply hearing advice, as if the idea that there *are* solutions is itself soothing. As if the advice proves that others care.

On the Front Lines

In early March, Penny learns from a coworker that the grounds department is redesigning some gardens next to the music building. Penny walks across campus and takes a look. A couple of groundskeepers are standing around studying an area of trees and rocks. A foreman says he wants to get rid of the rocks.

"Some of these are really nice rocks," Penny says.

They are dark gray, dappled with green and silver lichen.

"What, you want me to take a load of them to your house?" the worker jokes.

"Yeah!" Penny pauses, considering. "No, seriously, can I come and take some?"

The man grunts his assent. Twice during the following week Penny drives her car down the lane by the arts center after work, pries up boulders with a crowbar, and heaves them into the back of her little SUV. She piles them in the south corner of her yard. Afterward she's sore.

The plant nerd decides to spend a weekend at a conference on rock gardens. She calls her sister Sophie, who agrees to drive north and stay the weekend with their mom. It will be Penny's vacation, time away from the television and doctors' appointments and medications and overseeing home health aides. She is lucky to get away (so many caregivers don't have the chance), but the respite doesn't come free. Knowing she will leave on Friday, she roasts a chicken on Wednesday, cuts the meat off the bone, stores it in the refrigerator. She saves the bones and simmers stock. She makes corned beef and cabbage. She takes her mother out to lunch at a prime-rib place nearby, in part because Penny can take leftovers home for the weekend. The fridge fills.

Penny amasses food, she says, because her sister "uses her smoke alarm as a timer when she cooks. That's a joke, obviously, but it's based on some fact and observation." Penny giggles. She feels the closest to Sophie of all her siblings. "I'm my mom's best advocate, and Sophie is *my* best advocate." Sophie visits a couple of times a month and sometimes takes Mary to her house for a few days, to spell Penny. Penny's other sister, Deborah, stops by monthly and balances Mary's checkbook. Penny sees one of her two brothers a few times a year. The other she sees the least of all her siblings. He has dropped in for visits to Mary unannounced, and this bothers Penny. He and Penny have trouble getting along.

Penny is grateful for Sophie's help, but as with many family caregivers, siblings are in general a source of frustration. In Penny's case, she sees four people with, theoretically, the same obligations, yet they are maddeningly removed from Penny's day-to-day struggles with Mary. Penny remembers Sophie saying, "Well, you're probably the best qualified" to take care of Mom "because of your hospice training." Penny says, smiling, "It's like 'Shut up. Yeah, right.' That's because she didn't want to do it."

"Did you feel like you didn't want to do it, but you would?" I ask.

"No. I didn't feel like I didn't want to do it. I felt like it was the right thing to do."

．．．

Inga is another of Penny's best advocates. Inga, who sees caregiving as "doing what's necessary out of love and compassion," met Penny when Penny showed up at a group meeting in early 2009. Inga had been attending for three months. She listened to Penny's story about taking her mother in, to Penny's complaints that she felt unsupported by her siblings, and Inga felt empathy. She had tended not just Louise, her partner, but her grandmother, mother, and daughter. Listening to Penny, Inga thought mostly of her own mother. "Everything I heard, it reminded me of what I'd been through," she says. "I thought, 'I can support this woman.'" Inga wanted Penny to know, for instance, that Penny's siblings' reactions around their mother's care "have more to do with them than with you." She encouraged Penny to strive for detachment. Inga thought she could be "a good listener" for Penny. Maybe Inga could "say the kinds of things that I would have wanted to hear."

Believing that "you need to help and support and urge one another through this life," she hosted Penny, Mary, and Sophie for brunch one weekend. After that, having heard that Mary loves classical music, Inga kept Penny posted about local concerts. "Do with your mother," she told Penny, "what you can, while you can. You'll feel good about it later." Sometimes the two "couples"—Inga and Louise, Mary and Penny—ran into each other at concerts. As the months went on, Penny shared her anger with Inga, who thought, "I might be able to speak to Penny on behalf of Mary." She found herself "distressed" about Penny's anger. It's understandable, Inga says. But "it's going to be unproductive.'"

Of Inga, Penny says, "She's a friend, and she's not going to let go. She gives me a hug and there's just this *transfer* of energy." In coming months, Penny will rely on Inga to help steady her when things get rough.

• • •

Like other caregivers, Penny has taken on multiple roles. She tends not just to Mary's private bodily functions, her physical safety, her moods. She is also the manager of Mary's more public life as a patient. Penny keeps track of medications, doctors' appointments, diagnoses. She oversees home health aides. She watches over finances and strategizes about how care will get paid for in the months and years to come. As she does this work in the marketplace, she is also a patient advocate. She works to ensure for Mary the best possible care within a complicated medical system.

"When she reached the coverage gap," Penny tells the group this winter, "we started getting notices" from Medicare. This year, 2010, under cost-cutting limits that Medicare has placed on prescription-drug benefits, some patients must pay entirely for their medications for part of the year; these people are said to be in "the donut hole" until benefits start up again. (Two years later, President Obama will announce a phasing out of the donut hole.) Even the federal government uses the bakery term on its websites.

Penny dislikes it. Why not "coverage gap"? she wonders. "That's what it is."

She tells everyone about her latest efforts in keeping track of her mother's needs, diagnoses, conditions, appointments—and how she gets them paid for. Mary receives a pension from the VA because John Jessup served in the army. Penny faxed the VA a report of Mary's expenses, called later to check on it, and the staff person on the phone said she hadn't received the fax.

"I'm thinking, 'Goddang them,'" Penny says, looking around the table. "You really have to stay on top of these people."

"You truly are a case manager," Ben says.

"You know, I'm thinking that's true. The other day I was asking all these questions, and this guy said, 'Are you a doctor?'"

"'No,' I said.

"'Are you a nurse?' he asked.

"'No,' I said. I wanted to say"—she smiles—"'I'm just a smart-ass!'"

The first time Penny and I got together outside the support group, she said of her caregiving, "I'm on the front lines." It's a military analogy that, given her plant nerd's attention to detail, and a certain fierceness, seems apt. One day she tells the group about taking Mary to the "memory" clinic. The receptionist was new. Penny and her mother arrived at four fifteen for their appointment.

The receptionist looked up. "Your appointment was changed to three p.m."

"No one told me that," Penny said.

"I talked to your mother. I gave her the message."

Penny thought, And where is it you work again? The *memory* clinic?

The receptionist said, "I told her to write it down!"

Penny smiles, telling the story. "Does she not know where she works? With people with *Alzheimer's*! My mother said, 'If she'd called, I would have written it down!' Well, you can't blame my mom. She's the one with the disease!" Group members shake their heads.

Support-group meetings often become empowerment sessions. Penny and others do combat in the rough terrain of health-care bureaucracy—tracking details, forms, phone calls, specialists' opinions. Penny intervenes between her mother and a system on which her mother depends. Penny deals with doctors, nurses, nursing assistants, office workers—some of whom may be cranky, distracted, incompetent, perhaps beleaguered, themselves. These people, Penny seems to feel, must be *watched*.

An occasional group member says, "You're counting on these professional people. You're at their mercy." Caregivers negotiate with these "professional people" in all sorts of settings: in hospitals ("I would like you first to consult with his primary-care doctor"), in physicians' offices ("Could you explain why you made this diagnosis?"), nursing homes ("I do not want him taken to the hospital"), assisted-living facilities ("I believe my mother needs to be more active"). Group members' tactics differ according to their personalities, backgrounds, circumstances, and generations. Some, usually older, caregivers accept medical professionals' views without question, having all their lives seen doctors as high authorities. Others adopt technical language to earn respect. One member's chronicle for doctors of her own health problems, for example, will include the line "Symptoms worsen with ambulation." The phrase seems more powerful, perhaps, than "I feel worse when I walk."

Even the word *caregiver* is a technical, postindustrial, postfeminist, *public* term—necessary only in societies in which caring for our old and dependent is no longer conscripted by family roles. In preindustrial societies, the words *wife, daughter,* and *daughter-in-law* (and less often *son* and *husband*) sufficed, and in many parts of the world, still do. In twenty-first-century America, health care has become a commodity, to be purchased in a marketplace—although often the usual rules of the market do not apply. Health care and its roles have also been bureaucratized, made impersonal. It may be extreme, but still useful, to say, no longer is a *person* cared for, but a body and its organs managed by a (partially) market-driven system—with the caregiver as public-private go-between.

Penny's military analogy could be extended: she is on the front lines, protecting civilians—her mother—by battling an impersonal system that, she hopes, ironically, will help keep Mary alive.

The care that the system delivers does save many lives and

enables many people to live much longer than they otherwise would. Still, navigating the system, trying to get a loved one's needs met, can feel, and even become, adversarial. Penny's chief weapon in this battle is "The Golden Notebook"—an eleven-by-seventeen-inch volume with a metallic cover that lives on her kitchen table. In it she records episodes in Mary's care. She started writing in August of 2006. Three and a half years later, the thick book is filled with entries and dates and occasional doodles. On the cover she has stuck a note for the home health aides: "PLEASE sign in (name, date) & leave a note . . . How's the mommy doing? Thank you!" Still, most of the jottings on Mary's care are in Penny's handwriting.

Overseeing paid help at home also falls to the family care-giver, the unpaid care manager. Penny is the de facto supervisor, watching over the aides—although in this case, technically, they are employed by their agencies (to which Penny, using Mary's account, writes checks every month). One day an aide forgets about Mary's dentist appointment. The dentist's office calls Penny at work. Penny leaves work, drives home, and takes her mother herself. Penny finds out that a different aide is going to Boston that weekend to see her boyfriend, who is getting out of *jail*. This makes Penny feel just a little uncomfortable. Over the coming year, the Monday-Wednesday-Friday aide will turn over four times. In two of these cases Penny will ask the agency to have her replaced. One of the aides, Penny will find out from her police-officer neighbor, was once arrested herself—by him—for fighting.

Penny says to the group, "I'm thinking, 'What's wrong with our country that people with low skills and little education are tak-ing care of our kids and our old people? And the people who can swing a bat make a million dollars?'"

• • •

Certainly the need for well-trained, caring home health aides is growing fast. Home health workers are in ever-more demand in part because many of the increasing population of frail elders need only a few hours a day of home care; more intensive, expensive, twenty-four-hour institutional care is unnecessary. State governments are also increasingly looking to encourage this sort of limited and less costly care over stays in nursing facilities. State policies have been influenced, too, by a 1999 decision by the US Supreme Court that ruled that disabled people have the right to be cared for in the least-restrictive settings possible. The elderly also, of course, often prefer to remain and be helped in their homes.

Penny is right that direct-care workers receive little pay and are less educated than the American population generally. They struggle with poor working conditions. Only recently have they won the most basic labor rights. They must often work unpredictable hours. They make considerably less than the median American wage and usually work part-time, even when they'd like to work full-time. Almost half receive incomes less than twice the federal poverty rate, qualifying them for Medicaid and food stamps. Most do not have health insurance. More than half either possess only a high school degree or did not finish high school.

While advocates and many state governments are trying to improve formal home care, the system's low wages and poor working conditions have frequently meant high turnover and a workforce that is less than ideally prepared. Caregivers like Penny often pick up the slack.

I find a passage on the website of the Family Caregiver Alliance that describes Penny's care-coordination role from a broad perspective. Our health-care system deals best with acute health emergencies, the passage says. The system responds less well to the multiple, chronic, interrelated health problems that tend to develop in old age. The old often visit many doctors a year, "receive duplicate tests and procedures, [conflicting] diagnoses for the same set of symptoms, and contradictory medical information." Family caregivers often oversee all this care. Caregivers deal with many of the tasks that are considered nonmedical but that nevertheless are essential to their charges' survival—managing medications, dealing with transitions in and out of the hospital, and helping at home—all with little assistance and training.

I e-mail the passage to Penny. She writes back with the latest frustration: She had made an appointment with her mother's primary-care doctor. The office had rescheduled the appointment, and Penny had forgotten to put the new time on the calendar. The office had not called with a reminder, which Penny had come to expect—"too little staff and time, so they eliminated this service," Penny writes—and Mary missed her appointment. Penny had to reschedule the appointment for a later time, delaying Mary's care.

Meanwhile in Washington, health-care reform has stumbled along. Around the time I e-mailed that passage to Penny, in March of 2010, President Obama signed the Patient Protection and Affordable Care Act, designed to increase access to health insurance and provide patient protections. Measures relevant to elder caregiving included "care coordination for older adults" and a "person-centered approach" to managing multiple conditions. The law seeks to encourage the development of "patient-centered medical homes" as an approach to primary care, in which a team of health-care staff, led by a primary-care physician, coordinates patients' care. The central aims of medical homes are to provide better, more effective care and reduce costs. The approach's emphasis on care coordination for patients with multiple health problems may relieve some of the burden felt by family caregivers.

Another important element in elder caregiving is planning for end-of-life care. A provision in the health-care reform bill before it was passed required that doctors be reimbursed by Medicare for speaking with their terminally ill patients about their wishes for end-of-life care. Physicians might have asked, for example, which lifesaving medical measures a patient would want, and at what point a patient would prefer only comfort care. A doctor might also simply have asked after a patient's worries and priorities. But conservatives in Congress conducted a public-relations campaign against this part of the health-care reform bill, saying the requirement would create "death panels," and charging that doctors would have the power to decide whether an ill and/or elderly person should continue life-prolonging treatments—or be required to die. The "death panel" argument had the desired effect: the provision was removed.

In Massachusetts in 2010, a law similar to Obama's reforms was already in effect. It required all residents to have health insurance and provided it or a subsidy to those who couldn't afford it. Almost all residents carried health insurance as a result. Later, in 2012, the state legislature and the governor would take on the "third rail" of health-care reform: lowering health-care costs. The state would pass a package of measures—similar to the federal law—that encourage the creation of "accountable care organizations." ACOs share similarities with medical homes, but extend the care-coordination network and responsibility to include specialists and hospitals. ACOs are rewarded for achieving results rather than for the number of procedures they perform. So in theory, primary-care doctors, specialists, and hospitals will work together to promote the health of patients, like Mary, who have long-term, interrelated, chronic problems that can lead to serious illnesses, hospitalizations—and higher costs.

Penny's "Golden Notebook" provides a case study of such complexly related, chronic troubles (although Mary's problems are mild compared to the money-draining, major illnesses of many seniors). Beginning in the fall of 2009, continuing through 2010 and into 2011, Penny will record interrelated concerns regarding Mary's health and consultations with several doctors: Mary's dementia, one doctor thinks, might be worsened by obstructive sleep apnea. The doctor orders a sleep study, which finds that Mary does have the condition, which means she isn't getting enough oxygen at night. So Penny learns how to help Mary use a CPAP mask. Mary's eye pressure rises to dangerous levels. Her heartbeat, always leisurely, has slowed to the point of real concern: thirty-eight beats a minute. This condition could be depriving her brain of oxygen, too, and may help explain why Mary is lethargic and reluctant to exercise. Her primary-care physician says that Aricept, one of Mary's memory medications, could be causing the low heart rate. So could her glaucoma medication, or the combination of the two. This doctor believes, however, that Mary should continue taking these medications. Meanwhile Mary has issues with her gums, an infection in her foot, and at one point tests high in a measure of how hard her heart is working—likely a result, it turns out, of high sodium in the Meals-On-Wheels that Penny has ordered for Mary several times a week. For each of many of these problems, she sees a different provider. It's up to Penny, in large part, to keep track of it all.

• • •

In seeking answers to medical problems, Penny is at once expectant and wary of health-care providers and agencies. She wonders, for instance, about the ethics of her mother's "memory" doctor, in whose office Penny sees products advertising Namenda and other Alzheimer's medications. The sight of brand names makes Penny uncomfortable, especially because their effectiveness is questionable at best. For Mary's heart-rate problem, Penny takes Mary to two cardiologists—first one and, months later, another at a hospital Penny prefers. Both cardiologists, at different times, ask Penny to help Mary wear a Holter monitor for a day. Penny wonders why the results of the first monitor couldn't have been passed from one practice to the other.

After the second monitor, Penny takes Mary back to the doctor to discuss the readings. Penny expects the cardiologist to be self-important, a trait she presumes in specialists. He turns out to have a sense of humor, which relieves her.

Penny tells him that another doctor has brought up the possibility of Mary's needing a pacemaker.

Mary interjects, "I *don't* need a pacemaker!"

The cardiologist turns playfully to Mary. "Oh! Are you a *doctor*? Where did you go to medical school?"

Later in the meeting, the doctor pauses in conversation. He sits and places his thumb tip to the middle finger of each hand, lays the backs of his hands on his knees, closes his eyes, and makes, ironically, as if to meditate.

"Wow," Penny says, smiling, and turning to her mother. "I think we upset him. I think he's trying to *relax*."

Penny finds herself relaxing, too. Later she tells the story to the group. "I was anticipating he'd act like a really big ego. Which maybe he has. But he was also nice."

• • •

Still, Penny finds it trying, this negotiation between her mother and the world of professional medicine. Most other members do, too. Through the winter months, many in the group have come to see Penny's notebook, the keeping of records, as a necessary weapon. When they refer to it, the words sound capitalized. Liz, whose husband has recently moved to a veterans home, says to the group, "I've started The Notebook. I have my questions" for staff, "and I write their answers. Then I can refer back and say, '*Well,* on February *sixth* you said . . .'"

"There's prejudice against caregivers," Rufus says as the meeting ends. Inga, William, and Penny are pushing back their chairs. "But it does appall me that so many are so passive. They're the people who have the responsibility, and who are going to have the heartache—"

"—and who don't have The Notebook!" Penny says, referring to those hypothetical less assertive caregivers. She stands and heads toward the door.

🌿 Home

William's wife, Joan, stops eating. A small mound of chicken salad still sits on her plate. She sighs, a brief sigh, but William has his radar on his wife, as always. "What's the matter?" William asks, leaning toward her. Joan puts her hands up to her face. "What's the matter?"

She mumbles, "I can't keep track of things."

This is, oddly, a moment of clarity; Joan sometimes surfaces in this way. More often she says to William, "I'm ready to go home now," although she never can.

She points to the dishes in the center of the table. William says, "Oh, those are just the dirty dishes, Joan. I'll take them away." William picks up a small, white bowl filled with purée. "Do you want this?" He lifts it to his nose and sniffs. "I think it's apple-sauce." He puts the dish in front of her and takes the others to the nurses' station.

Joan clutches the spoon. She scoops the sauce into her mouth and gums and swallows. William sits back down. Joan eats half of the purée, then reaches out a finger and scratches at the blue table-cloth. She says something unintelligible. "What's that?" William asks, turning toward her.

"What about this?" she asks slowly, moving her finger on the tablecloth next to the dish. William shakes his head, not under-standing. He shrugs and smiles at me.

I remember trying to understand my sons as babies. My brain toils in a like way, matching up clues. I say, "Maybe she wants the other dish taken away."

A moment later—perhaps the moment Joan's impaired brain takes to process what I've said—her face brightens, dark eyebrows lifting. She leans and punches William in the arm. "You're. Not as smart. As you think you are," she says in her labored way. She turns, surprisingly, and smiles a toothless smile at me. "Is he?"

The question could signal sisterly collusion ("*Oh,* those men!"), and maybe it does, but her expression is innocent, uncomplicated, as if she really wants to know just how smart this man is, and would I tell her? She smiles again, eyes twinkling, and leans in and punches William in the arm. Again.

William knows the support group admires his devotion, his daily visits to Joan. "I don't know what it is," he says. "A certain time of the day, I'll be doing something—like today I was going through papers—and about ten thirty, quarter of eleven, I say, 'Well, I gotta get ready to go.' It's something over here tells me to go." He taps his chest.

He wheels Joan slowly down the hall, leaning slightly on the handles of the wheelchair. She, in white socks and cream-colored slip-on shoes, holds her feet just above the floor as she's pushed along. On her floor live residents with dementia and without. The nurses and aides all know Joan. By the nurses' station, Carla, a young aide, says, "There's my girl! Let me say hi." William stops. Carla kneels in front of Joan and puts her hands on Joan's waist. "How are you?" Carla says, staring into Joan's eyes.

"Good," Joan says, her blue eyes looking back.

"Very good!" Carla has blond hair pulled into a ponytail, hoop earrings so large that they brush her shoulders.

"Very good," Joan murmurs.

William wheels on. He tells me the names of some of the residents along the hall. He points into a room. "There's a woman who has just turned one hundred." At a turn in the loop of hallway, the smell turns from old-person sweet—not exactly pleasant but not offensive either—to a smell of feces. The place seems clean, though. Each room has two beds. Bob, a large, bald man with gnarled, arthritic hands, sits in a wheelchair in the doorway to a lounge. A television plays a game show. He sees Joan and smiles, lifting one hand from its rest.

"We'll stop and say hi," William says to Bob. He parks Joan next to and facing Bob. She reaches for Bob's hand. He takes it eagerly. He has a round, toddler face. "You're good," he says, looking at Joan's face. "You're very good." Joan strokes his hand with her free one. "You're so nice. You're so nice." Tears brim in his eyes.

"Oh, Bob, don't cry," an aide says. She's been watching from behind William.

Bob's wife had been here, too, for rehab, but had gone home. "Are you going to go home, too?" William says.

Bob nods and looks down.

"Okay. We'll come back around and say hi again." William inches the wheelchair back, causing Joan's hand to relinquish Bob's.

In Joan's room William has smoothed an institutional blue spread over her low hospital bed. He's arranged stuffed bears that crowd a shelf above the headboard. He pulls a plastic photo album from the shelf and shows me pictures—a boat he owned; Joan, not long before she became ill, with their motor home in Florida; Joan with her mother, who was then in a wheelchair with Alzheimer's. At the back of the album he's placed photos he wants to show me: the cake Joan made for a friend's wedding, multilayered, bridges from a center cake to satellite ones, all in lacy frosting and embellishments. It looks professional. She made cakes for friends and family, charging them only for the ingredients. "Joan liked to help people out. That was her thing." William points to another photo, of baskets she'd made, evenly crafted and sturdy. Joan sits by us in her wheelchair as William talks, perhaps listening.

Back in the hall, William notices Joan's dangling shoe, kneels, and wriggles it back on. "Is that better?"

"I guess," Joan says.

"There's the lunch cart, Joan," William says. A young man wheels a big metal box down the hall. "Let's go get the towels." From a closet near the nurses' station, he grabs a small stack of white terry-cloth bibs. He plops the stack onto Joan's lap. "Let's go hand them out." He turns to me. "It's something to do," a part of their routine.

In the small dining room, opposite the aides' station, a staff member turns on a CD player. "Boogie Woogie Bugle Boy" fills the room. William wheels Joan up to a table, draws up chairs for me and for himself. A drooping woman with wispy, white hair, nearly bald, hunches in a wheelchair, waiting for her food. "This is Eva," William says. "She'll talk our ear off."

"Oh!" Eva says, straightening a little and peering brightly up at William. "You know who I am! Who are you?"

"I'm William."

"Do you live on East Street?"

"No, I live in Burton."

"Oh!" She names a man she knows there. "Do you know him?"

"Oh, yes, I know him. He's the fire chief."

"He's very nice." Eva points at Joan. "Is she your wife?"

"Yes."

William has already sat at lunch many times with Eva.

A nursing assistant sets a tray with a chicken-salad sandwich and a styrofoam cup labeled MAGIC CUP and FORTIFIED in front of Eva. On Joan's tray is a plate with chicken salad, pureed broccoli, a small white roll, mashed potatoes. William takes a roll, tears and butters it, puts it back in front of Joan. He opens Joan's carton of milk and places it in front of her. She sits blankly. "Come on, you need to eat," he says. He scoops a forkful of chicken salad and moves it toward her mouth. It opens, and she chews.

"I never thought I'd be doing this," William says, shaking his head. He probably includes family finances, housework, yard work—keeping track of everything.

After a few mouthfuls, Joan grasps the spoon herself. She stares, mostly at nothing. She eyes me occasionally. She eats sequentially from right to left, scooping everything in the path of her spoon. A bite, a glance at William, as if to reassure herself he is still there. A bite and then a stare at me, perhaps wondering who I am, because William usually comes alone and gives her all his attention.

An attendant wheels up another resident, Belle. Belle stoops even more than the others; she cannot lift her head. She must be fed. Carla, who attends her, is energetic. She sits between Belle and Eva, leans in close to Eva's face, and says, *"Babka."* Eva says something back. "She's teaching me Polish," Carla says to me. Eva leans toward Carla and says something more. "What's that mean?" Carla says.

"I'm looking for a boyfriend!" Eva says, and chuckles.

Eva is both sharp and easily confused. "My birthday is October eighth, 1910—or something." This year she'll turn one hundred, if she makes it that far.

Joan's behavior has been fine since she moved here, William says. No catastrophes—although "she is feisty."

"She's feisty," Carla echoes, spooning another bite toward Belle, "but she's a love bug."

Carla and the other aides seem affectionate, caring. Yet I will walk these halls at other times, when William is not around, and the place will seem more bleak. Residents sit blankly in wheelchairs, queued up along the walls. The line between compassionate, engaging care and benign neglect—perhaps worse—often seems thin in nursing homes. William's presence helps secure the line, perhaps not just because he is a witness, a watchful presence, but because he provides the staff with help—and company. Several have become his friends.

Another aide calls from across the small dining room that Joan "was up early this morning. I got her up and we went right to the shower."

"Did she bite you?" William asks.

"No! She was good. I knew it was going to be a good day."

Carla says she had gone up to Maine for the weekend with a friend. The friend's brother had a pig. Carla leans close again to ninety-nine-year-old Eva, Polish instructor, who has been taking a bite of sandwich, then a bite of orange ice cream, then a bite of sandwich, methodically. "I saw a three-hundred-pound pig over the weekend. Did you ever have a pig?"

"Oh, yes," Eva says. "We had pigs and cows and turkeys."

"Did you ever have a *three-hundred-pound* pig?"

"Oh, I don't know. I think more like two-fifty," Eva says. That is the usual size for butchering. Eva still remembers her farm facts. "Are they going to kill it?"

"Well, yes, eventually," Carla says with an apologetic look.

"They usually do," Eva says matter-of-factly. She takes another tiny bite of sandwich.

Joan has slowly excavated her way across the piles on her plate, chewing, her cheeks folding and buckling. William says he is about to drive back down to Cape Cod. His friend Roger will come along and help with some heavy lifting. There is a chimney to fix. In early May he will go along with "the girls" from the nursing home down to a casino in Connecticut. "It's not really my thing. But it's something new to do."

The music, still tunes from the forties, turns lugubrious. The man at the next table, William whispers, has cancer. The man is missing an ear; his eye weeps blood. Carla walks over and rubs the man's bald head. "You got a haircut?" she asks, smiling. He mutters something. William says the man likes to arm-wrestle with him and is still strong.

"Does it depress you to come here?" I ask William.

"Now I'm used to people like this. I get to know them. Who they are. Their names. When Joan's mother was in the nursing home, I hated to go there." William shakes his head. "But not anymore." He knows, he will tell the support group, that visits to Joan help him, too. He feels valued, connected. He appreciates his friendships with "the girls," and visiting every day must result in Joan's getting better care.

Eva has polished off her lunch. "Are you going to stay here tonight?" she asks William.

"No, I'm going home."

"Do you live on East Street?"

"No, I live in Burton."

"Oh. Are you going to stay here tonight?"

"No," William says. "I'm going home."

PART II

SPRING

Assisted Living

Hothouse

Every March, the college where Penny works hosts a flowering-bulb show in one of its greenhouses. Sweet-scented tulips, daffodils, and other narcissi exult under a vaulted glass roof that is all sky, offering warmth and color a few weeks before the outside world does. Winter-weary New Englanders converge on the campus, snap pictures, and lean over blooms, inhaling. On the Friday evening of the show's first weekend, a speaker inaugurates the event with a keynote lecture. This year Penny drives home from work before the lecture, picks up Mary, and drives her back. She escorts her mother to the lecture hall in the student center. A botanical designer from New York clicks through slides of Central Park. She talks about cultivating beauty, plants, and nature in public spaces—the power of landscape to give solace, build community, and promote calm in tough places.

Afterward the audience chats and files out. I greet Mary, who has a broad smile and lively eyes. Penny helps Mary wrestle into a black winter coat. Mary steps toward the hall's entrance, wielding her walker with a kind of authority. She turns it, shifts herself into alignment with it, shoves it forward, and glides out of the room. We head toward the elevator. She says to Penny, in what seems like a bid to entertain me, "You never take me *anywhere*."

Penny laughs. We wait for the elevator. Penny tells a story: In a department store, Mary spied a stocking trailing from a woman's pant leg. Mary placed her foot on the stocking; the woman kept walking. The stocking slid from the woman's pant leg. The woman looked down, noticed, reached, and hurriedly stuffed the stocking into her purse. She glared at Mary, stomped away. "Mom was pleased with herself. She figured she'd caught a woman shoplifting. But who knows," Penny says, laughing, "maybe it was just stuck in her pants from the day before!" The elevator doors slide open, and Mary pushes forward, chuckling.

Penny asks me to stand with Mary by the glass doors at the front of the student center while Penny gets the car. Mary sighs, re-aims her walker, and sits on its folding seat. "I like to tease her," she says. "It's just what I do."

Mary is charming. She seems sharp, engaged. How could this be? But I'm learning. Personality persists, social skills linger, even after memory fades. This seems particularly true for Mary. At once testy and graceful, she is cheerful, but also knows how to complain poignantly. Making conversation as we wait, I ask her about her days. "I watch television," she says. "It's all I do. What else *can* I do?"

Back in 2007, Mary's neurologist had diagnosed her with mild cognitive impairment. Another doctor later diagnosed vascular dementia. Still later, a clinician called Mary's dementia "probable Alzheimer's." Dementia diagnosis is inexact. Penny did not trust the last doctor—the one whose office is strewn with drug-company brand names—and ignored her opinion. If Mary's dementia *is* vascular, her memory loss is caused by multiple small strokes in her brain—so small that they did not produce obvious symptoms at the time they occurred. They would have, though, caused such loss of communication among brain cells that now, Penny says, "her short-term memory is completely shot." Mary has great difficulty with short-term, "episodic" memory—with remembering plans, who called earlier in the day, or whether she has eaten lunch.

With dementia, as the brain becomes more diseased, other forms of memory go, too. Even the most mundane tasks become impossible. Consider the simple duty of brushing your teeth. You need memory for every step: You remember to do it. You remember where the bathroom is, where you keep the toothpaste and brush. You remember how to open the cabinet, grasp the toothbrush, run the water, spread toothpaste, move the brush over your teeth. You look in the mirror and recognize yourself. You recall associations about yourself, the ideas that form your sense of self, who you are. You remember, without even realizing it, there is *I*.

Imagine hearing, as you stand in the bathroom, a knock on the door. Without effort, you remember who'd been in the house with you when you stepped into the bathroom. You casually say hello to your spouse.

Your memory has served, and in various ways: you have used long-term, "implicit" memory—how to brush your teeth—and long-term autobiographical memory—you remember your spouse. Now imagine that your spouse tells you that you have an appointment scheduled for three hours later. Your brain must process this information and "store" it, to be retrieved as the hours pass, so that you remember to keep your appointment. This is where Mary's memory most often fails her—and it is the form of memory that most commonly declines first as people age, and/or as dementia develops.

Memory is so central to functioning—from physical tasks that use unconscious memory, to memory that is central to identity, such as recognizing loved ones—that as it slowly declines, a person's competence, her selfhood, even what we may see as her humanness, slowly fades away. With Alzheimer's disease, memory used for the most basic functions—walking, speaking, swallowing, even digesting—disintegrates. The disease kills its sufferers—

unless something else causes death first—because the brain can no longer remember how to keep them alive.

In mid-March, a new woman arrives in the support group, accompanied by her sister. Sarah and Bridget have similar broad, ruddy faces. They sit close to each other, comfortably. Ben asks Sarah to introduce herself. She describes her situation. Before long she is weeping. "My husband has early Alzheimer's, and I'm having a hard time managing myself." He was diagnosed a couple of years ago. "Friends saw it coming. At first I was in denial," she says. "Now I'm rageful." She has had a rewarding career as a psychiatric nurse. "I've taken care of people all my life." She looks around the table at others who have already spoken. "I took care of your wife," she says to William. "And *your* wife," she says to Daniel. She means this figuratively. Yet, despite this professional experience, caring for her husband feels like more than she can handle.

"I'm very depressed," she says. A few years before, a violent patient had injured Sarah's arm. She had to go on disability. She is not handling the loss of her work well, she says. She volunteers at the town's senior center to feel useful. "I get angry at my husband" for his growing disabilities. "Walter was a cop in the sixties. A drug-busting cop, the Archie Bunker of the department, a forensic photographer. He took photos of suicides, murders. It was a horrible career, in terms of what he was exposed to." Sarah turns and looks at her sister. "He was macho, right?" Bridget nods. Now he can't remember how to use a can opener. "He works at Stop and Shop," pushing shopping carts and loading groceries into sacks. "He likes to brag about being the oldest bag boy." Sarah smiles through tears. The job, she says, gives him purpose. He is earning money; he feels useful. She worries about the day when he'll have to give it up. Looking around the table, she says she also wonders how often he "puts a ten-pound ham on top of your dozen eggs."

Ben asks if Walter is aware of his diagnosis. "Not really," Sarah says. He has other problems that preoccupy him—a bad hip and back. "He's more focused on his physical pain."

"Is he angry?" Ben asks.

"No."

"No," Bridget echoes. "*She's* angry."

"You wait all your life for your golden years and—" Sarah cuts herself off. "I'm really ticked off."

Group members have been listening attentively. Ben says, "Thank you."

Later, at the end of the meeting, Ben turns again to Sarah. "The progressive nature of the disease is hard. Keep us posted."

Sarah nods. "I'll be here every week. I've already decided."

An occasional member, Miriam, speaks up. For eleven years, Miriam cared fiercely for her husband, James, through Parkinson's and Lewy body dementia. He died a few months ago. ("Incidentally," she tells the group once, "this was not my plan. I kept him at home for all those years because I was going to stand between him and death.") She returns to the group now as "the caregiver of Miriam."

Today she asks, "Sarah, do you have a professional listener? A therapist?"

"I have my *sister*," Sarah says, leaning toward Bridget.

"But she's not a professional," Miriam says, shaking her head. Miriam wears red cat-eye glasses, her long gray hair in a topknot. "You're *grieving* right now. That's so hard because he's right there in front of you."

Sarah nods and wipes tears with a paper napkin from the table. She smiles and says, "I hope the group isn't like this every week!"

• • •

It usually isn't. Ben will look back on Sarah's arrival and say, "Sarah brought the gift of affect to the group," his social-worker reference to her open expression of emotion. More "affect" has slowly surfaced in meetings over the years, from the men's relative stoicism, their World War II conversations, through the arrival of Liz, Miriam, Inga, Penny. But up to Sarah's arrival, Ben says, "I didn't even think about the fact that we needed tissues. That day, we had this big, lunky napkin container on the table. I kind of dumped it in front of her." Sarah's arrival "represented a turning point," he says. "The group opened up." Soon "people were bringing in these nice, juicy, angry stories."

Ben never will supply tissues. People get used to pushing the napkin container across the table whenever someone cries.

In April, an elderly couple, Karen and Don, take seats at the conference table. Sarah tells them they look familiar. She realizes she has met them at the senior center. In this small city, paths cross often. Karen had called Ben before the meeting and said that she needed to bring Don along. He couldn't stay home alone. Ben welcomes them both.

Don, pale-eyed, bald, and slender, says, "I'm the care*taker*." He points toward Karen to his right. "She's the *giver*."

Karen nods tersely. She says she'll just listen today. "We have some problems. I thought I'd be able to handle the anger"—she gestures her head toward Don—"but I'm not."

For the next several months, Karen will sit through most meetings silently, an expression of bemused irritation on her face: lips pursed, a puzzled look. Don is happy to talk. He seems to be in the early stages of dementia (although Karen tells me privately that Don has not been diagnosed). He seems lucid, is a good talker, and still has capacity for insight. He says he has always been compe-

90

tent, a leader; "I have an aversion to thinking of myself as having to be taken care of." Yet, his impairments show: at each meeting, he repeats the same autobiographical material, his heroic experiences in World War II, his decades running a children's camp. He seems to be fighting to hold on to his sense of self, his dignity. His struggle, and his wife's dismay, is wearing at their marriage. At one spring meeting he says, "I know that I'm a very good manager." He makes a small motion toward Karen. "I just can't stand her"—he pauses—"aggressiveness."

Karen listens, lips pressed.

"I love her," Don says. "But she does lousy things."

"It's the hardest thing," Ben says, steering the conversation in a new direction. "We talk a lot about this upstairs"—he means in his behavioral health unit. "The dialectics of relationships. Situations where you love somebody so much, but they drive you bananas."

"If you didn't love her," Penny agrees, "you wouldn't be so pissed off."

"You love somebody," Ben says, "but you hate some of the things they do." The trick is "to metabolize those two opposing things. It's easier if you *don't* love them. You just write them off."

Penny leans toward Don. "Do you think there's some fear involved here, too?"

Don seems so capable of insight. "I never thought of myself as afraid of anything. I've done things that the average person couldn't dream of doing. I flew B-24s. Forty-seven missions. My last mission, I brought it home, crashed, a couple of guys dying. I had to get them home."

Ben nods. "How old are you now, Don?"

"Eighty-eight. I go to the senior center, and I can't find anybody who knows how to play pool like I do. I trounce everybody there."

Ben raises his eyebrows. "*Trounce?* That's a lonely place to be."

As the group's leader, Ben walks a fine line. It is not his job to get Don or Karen to change. His aim, he says, is to help provide them—Karen, really—with a place for support and idea sharing. To this end, he says, he tries to "generalize" issues that come up for individuals—to find ways that particular problems can be shared and discussed in productive ways. In the most basic sense, his job is simply to enable conversation. He turns to Karen. "You're looking like you'd like to say a few things."

Karen has short, sparse curls; she's wearing a sweatshirt, glasses on a chain around her neck. She has been sitting quietly, the same complicated expression on her face. "He doesn't remember anything. He denies—" She stops.

"Yeah. It sounds like Don can't see that part, and you can."

Don says, "It's the way she handles it," nodding toward his wife.

"Well," Penny says, "nobody can handle that stuff very well. A *saint* can't handle it well."

🌿 Life of Job

Each time Liz and Joe circle back through the empty waiting room, the television delivers a new message. Most of the time, Liz ignores the chatter, her eyes looking ahead. On round six or so, she glances up at the screen. A meteorologist points to a map. It is cold for an April morning. "Thirty-two in Millfield," Liz says. "Sheesh."

Four or five times every week, Liz walks around in circles at the veterans home with her husband. On nice days they walk outside, four times around the facility. Three times, Liz knows, makes a mile. Good exercise. But today the wind drives steely clouds across the valley, and Liz, who is sixty-two, has brought only her lightweight, pink jacket. Her auburn hair is neatly styled. "I thought we'd walk inside today," she has said to Joe. They step briskly along a narrow corridor, around a corner, down another hall, through the empty waiting room, back along the original corridor and around again. Historical pictures of men and women in medical uniforms hang on the white hospital walls.

There is formality to the players in the scene. Joe, seventy-four, small and trim, with glasses and closely shorn gray hair, his gait quick and rocking, pauses at each doorway and makes sure that Liz and I pass through first. Liz looks straight ahead, pocketbook in hand. Referring to her temperament, she says once to her support group with a wry smile, "I *have* been known to say the F-word." She is both decorous and flinty. Her trials have left her at once downtrodden and wryly steeled, not quite bitter but often turning to irony to mute the pain. *"Fa la la la la,"* she will say flatly to me at the end of the year, just before Christmas, after telling me that her son's middle-aged friend has just had a heart attack.

Behind us ambles Clint, tall, gray-haired, in a cap with military iron-on badges all over it. A volunteer and a veteran, he has accompanied Joe and Liz on these walks every Wednesday for weeks. Liz isn't sure why, beyond knowing Clint wants to do something good in his new retirement.

"What do you think of our facility here?" Joe asks me.

I glance at him. His face has a kind of distracted eagerness, a need to please. "I like it fine," I say. "What do you think of it?"

"Oh, I'm happy here. Happy as a clam." We turn a corner. Next corridor.

"It's nice to hear you say that," Liz says. "I think maybe you're just saying what you think we want to hear."

"Just like in the military!" Clint says, and chuckles.

Joe doesn't seem to get the joke. He says he watched a movie last night, *The Alamo* with John Wayne. "It was good."

Joe and Clint talk about the real Alamo; Clint says he went there during basic training down in Texas. Around and around, quick steps, Liz holding her pocketbook as if on errands. Joe says, "Well, I have a lot of videos." Liz buys them, usually out of big bins at Walmart.

I ask Joe with whom he watches the videos. "With Jacob," Joe answers. "He's a nice guy. He's a good conversationalist. He tells stories about growing up in Brooklyn."

"There are a lot of nice guys on the unit," Liz says, helping the conversation along.

"Yeah. There aren't too many fights. When there are, they have to call a time-out so they can take out the wounded," Joe says, deadpan. Later Liz will say, "Joe still has his sense of humor!"

On perhaps the fifteenth time around the loop, the television in the empty waiting room plays an ad for a funeral home. "A life well lived is a life worth remembering!" a woman chirps. Around the corner, back into the corridor, Joe asks me again, "What do you think of our facility here?" Same personable intonation, same exact words.

Earlier, I had climbed the stairs with Liz to Joe's small room. Opposite a low bed, heavy curtains shrouded a window; along one wall, lockers held a few of Joe's possessions. Joe wasn't there.

He arrived in the doorway. He seemed to be trying to appear normal. He also seemed confused. The two go together, the lostness and the effort at presence. Joe is still walking the long edge between awareness and oblivion.

"This is Nell," Liz said.

He shook my hand. "Hi, Mel."

"No, Nell," Liz said.

"Oh! Nell!" Joe said, shaking his head. Silly him.

People do indeed mishear that consonant. But Joe appears alert to the meaning of his missteps and is ready to apologize.

Mostly he comes across as a pleasant, cordial, if ill at ease, physically fit older man. If I hadn't known of his dementia, I wouldn't have recognized it, at first. Repeated questions, topics that circle back again, and again—they slowly become apparent. Liz finds it galling that Joe can appear so normal, in these early stages of dementia, to occasional and brief visitors. He, like Mary, can still muster social skills, long after other memory fails. Penny says of her mother, "People meet her and think there's nothing wrong. I hate that. Sort of." This is Liz's experience, too. Friends, acquaintances, even the staff at Joe's facility, seem to question whether there is really anything wrong. In these transitional months, Liz has felt abandoned by old friends, who stopped calling her after Joe's transfer because they questioned the move. On his unit at the veterans home, Joe receives oversight and minimal care. He is free to go outside, and he roams the building as he wants during the day—so staff don't spend extended time with him. They emphasize how *well* Joe is doing. Joe and Liz meet monthly with the nurse-manager and a social worker and review his case. Joe walks into the room and says, "Good morning, ladies! How are you all doing today?"

"No wonder," Liz says, "they see him as so high-functioning."

Liz is the one who hears Joe repeat phrases over and over. He acts differently, she says, with her than with everyone else. She coped with his hostile, threatening behavior before he ended up here. She says no one acknowledges that Joe is being fed a handful of mood-altering meds each day. Liz feels guilty, and she feels alone.

Joe's repetitions test Liz's patience. The burden they imply sits on her shoulders all the time, even after she has gone home and paid bills, called her son, cooked herself dinner. Often she spends the rest of her day in bed, nursing her headache. Lately her neck hurts, too; she has gone to Dr. Connor, whom she had recommended to Daniel, and endured cortisone shots.

. . .

Not surprisingly, research shows that a caregiver's perception of the quality of her relationship with her spouse, before he or she becomes dependent, helps determine both the caregiver's sense of burden, and how long she endures before moving her spouse to an institution. For years Liz has both felt bad about her marriage and experienced great caregiving burden. She moved Joe to a facility quite early. But to say simply and clinically that Liz had "low relationship satisfaction," to use one report's language, would be to miss what she doesn't dare say to the group: that Joe was verbally abusive toward her for most of their marriage.

His hostility first showed up in the beginning of their marriage, Liz says, after her headaches had started, back when his memory was fine. She thinks he grew angry because she was debilitated, didn't have the time and energy he wanted from her. He "shot daggers" with his looks, threw things, called her stupid, a "horrible wife." Over time she began to believe him. She spent "a lot of time in the bedroom, crying."

Joe's outbursts grew as his dementia progressed. In 2009, when she joined the group, she told everyone only about his current behavior and attributed it to his emerging disease. The longer-term behavior she kept to herself and—later, after Joe was at a facility—mostly the gladness that he was gone. It is not a conventionally virtuous sentiment. And Joe, she tells me, grew *up* in this town. He is well liked, respected, seen as a "great guy." She is afraid no one will believe her, even her support group. She feels out of place among devoted, grieving spouses. She worries about being judged.

Still, going to the group helps her rise to the challenges of caregiving. Back in May 2009, a couple of months after joining, Liz told everyone a story: Her son and daughter-in-law, who live nearby, had visited. After they had gone, Liz and Joe had discovered a puddle of gas in the driveway. It must have leaked from Liz's son's car. Liz figured she'd call the fire department. But Joe grabbed a brush with a long handle and started scrubbing at the puddle. He grumbled and complained.

"It's not their fault," Liz said, defensive on behalf of her son.

"I *know* that!" Joe growled. He turned to Liz, wielding the long-handled brush. "Get out of here!" he snarled. "Get out of my sight! If you know what's good for you, you'll get out of here." Liz fled to the bedroom. That evening, cramps gripped her gut. The pain worsened through the night. In the morning, she dared ask Joe to take her to the doctor. He did, the doctor sent Liz to the hospital, and she was admitted with ischemic colitis.

After she had recovered and relayed the story, group members asked Liz whether there were guns in her house.

"Yes," she said. Joe used to hunt.

Get rid of them, the group said.

Ben gave Liz a phone number for the county's emergency psychiatric service, the same number that William had used on the last day that Joan was home. Ben said Liz could call the line if she felt threatened again. He told her what to expect should she call.

Liz would be glad, later, to have the information. Back at her house, she phoned a friend who also owned guns. She figured he would know what to do with Joe's. The friend came over while Joe was out and carted all the guns away—or so Liz thought.

🌿 Institutions

The forsythia bloom, lining the drab hospital grounds in yellow. In the beds next to the college greenhouses, hyacinth shoots push their way up out of damp soil. Penny starts seedlings on her sunny, enclosed porch—broccoli, eggplant. She spends every moment she can with her garden. April, so recently cold, surprises with seventy- and eighty-degree days. The trees still leafless, there is little shade and the sun feels hot. Penny rakes out beds, scoops up leaves and branches, and dumps them under the ash and the maples in the backyard—not woods, really, but enough trees so in the summer they screen the highway. A small stream runs through. She has stuck a pair of pink flamingos into the ground by the stream. She smiles, discovering native trout lilies emerging from the damp soil. Skunk cabbages push through the dead, brown leaves, brilliant green, as if drawn with a child's crayon.

Penny has been trying to get Mary to exercise, even just to get up from the couch and get her own pudding out of the fridge. Mary expects Penny to bring the pudding to her. Mary has, it seems, an ability to wear down all her well-meaning adversaries, not just Penny. "The Golden Notebook," from late 2008 into 2009, shows notes from therapists: Mary should keep a memory journal. Mary should do her leg exercises. Eventually such notes fall away. Per- haps the professionals' coverage ran out, but I imagine Mary, con- tentedly watching TV, smiling, resisting, until the providers pack up their clipboards and advice and go on to other jobs. Mary sits, ever noncompliant, Penny's "little Buddha."

Penny, these days, feels far from a buddha. One April week- end, she has a caregiving "meltdown." She calls Inga and shares her troubles; Inga listens. Penny says she is weary of the "water tor- ture" of living with her mother. "All she does, all the time, is eat, sleep, poop, and watch TV. It's hard to watch somebody just watch TV." Penny's not sure when the question of "putting" her mother somewhere—she hates that word, *put*—first came to stew in her mind. After a while, the idea is tossing around on active boil. She thinks about both ifs and whens. She feels guilt for anticipating moving her mom, and guilt for even considering it. She worries about how her siblings will react, whether they'll be supportive. For a few months, Inga has been suggesting looking at long-term-care facilities, "just so you know what your options are."

Penny had first visited a place in her neighborhood back in January, a "continuing care retirement community"—an increasingly common type of long-term care. A person moves in, healthy and independent, ratchets up to limited care as he or she becomes infirm, moves to "assisted living" when necessary, and finally to a nursing home—all on the same campus. Penny didn't know any of this when she arrived unannounced that day. She had a custodian show her around and asked staff if they liked their jobs and how long they had worked there. She spoke to the charge nurse. She tells her support group that the nurse was welcoming and offered good information. Penny walked around in the "independent living" building, the dining room, the various sitting rooms.

She says to the group, "I'm thinking, 'This is really nice. *I* may end up here!'"

Ben says his aunt checked herself into assisted living when mildly demented.

"That'll be me!" Penny says, and giggles.

Penny says, "Inga's going to kick my butt if I don't" get serious about visiting more places. "She's going to say, 'Okay, which ones did you look at since we last talked?' I'm going to say, 'Zeee-roh.'" In mid-April, Penny calls and arranges two more visits, for a Tuesday afternoon.

Inga and I go along. We all meet for lunch beforehand. Penny has taken the day off. In a pub in an old mill town, a five-minute drive from Penny's house, we sit by a window looking out onto a narrow street of brick-front stores. Penny and Mary eat here often. But Mary is at home, as usual, unaware of Penny's errands.

Penny leans her elbows on the table and says that when she calls nursing homes and other "long-term-care facilities" to get information, she always gets transferred to a marketing person. "That's who they put you on the phone with first." She doesn't want to talk with a marketing person. She wants to do research, not sign up. Talking to the marketing department feels like sending her mom off too soon. "I'm not ready to let her go." She will say this several times during the day. She also fears the marketing people. "If they're like car salesmen, God help 'em."

She is overwhelmed. More and more is being asked of her. Angie, Mary's longest-term home health aide, recently asked Penny to make a corsage. Angie would have to pay $40 otherwise. Penny agreed to the favor. Another item on her list. She missed her mammogram appointment a day ago; she simply forgot. In the morning she took Mary to a doctor's appointment.

A waitress comes by. We order. Penny and Inga discuss whether Mary could live in "independent living." Penny is trying to understand the various terms. "I think maybe she could be in independent living with assistance," as one program is called. "If we had a plan."

Inga is doubtful. "You have no idea how many things you do to enable her to live" at home. "You think ahead. You prevent problems. You put a lot of mental work into it. In independent living, she would really be on her own," Inga says. "You'll want your mother with you until you know that her situation at home has become dangerous."

Penny wonders how she will know, unless it is too late.

They discuss the differences between Inga's mom, years ago, and Mary. Inga's mother lived in assisted living for only three months. She fell and hit her head on a bedside table and didn't survive.

"My mom could be there for three or four years," Penny says.

The waitress brings food. Penny talks about her job, says she feels her efforts for her mother are taking more and more time away from work.

Inga leans forward and looks Penny in the eye. "Are you behind?"

"No."

"Is there anything big coming up that you won't be prepared for?"

"No."

Inga sits back. "Get rid of the guilt."

"But I was raised Catholic!"

"Get rid of the Catholic." Inga laughs. "I'm a tough therapist."

Penny tosses garden gloves, a gray cap, and a yoga mat into a cardboard box and shoves the box across the backseat of her car. I get in. The car has a standard shift, no CD player, a tape deck. Two out of three of the seat belts in the back don't work. I buckle into the good one. Penny drives southeast over a small, steep mountain. Inga is in the passenger's seat. The valley below is leafing out amid sweet spring sunshine. There is still a view through the trees.

On the other side of the mountain, Penny pulls onto the highway. We see the veterans home, up on the hill, where Joe, Liz's husband, lives. Probably he has just finished lunch in the "canteen," is working on crafts, or napping. Inga holds a folder of forms and checklists on nursing-home quality that she and Penny have printed off a Medicare site. The forms ask about appearance, living spaces, policies, safety. We take an exit into a suburban town. Rhododendrons line boulevards. Big brick houses are set back from the road. Penny says that, growing up, she always thought of this town as the place where rich people lived. For some reason, she remembers a story about her mother: Mary was raised Catholic, but was excommunicated—that is what her family called it, anyway—from the Church when she married Penny's father, a divorced Protestant. Many years later, in a hospital, Mary was waiting for surgery on her bleeding ulcer. Mary talked with a priest. She told him that she had raised five children, had worked to support her family, had stayed with her husband until the end.

"Don't think you haven't been a good Catholic," the priest said. The story sounds like relief, like redemption.

We turn into a landscaped drive.

The nursing home is housed in a low brick building. Its central entrance looks like a hotel's, as if bellhops and parking valets should be waiting. Inside, on the lobby's walls, staff have hung plaques with donors' names. Elevator music plays.

"Pretty nice," Penny says.

The place looks well funded. Penny will learn in a few moments, though, that most of its patients are far from wealthy. Lucy, the director of admissions, petite and wearing shiny black pumps, leads Penny, Inga, and me down a hall to a small sitting room. Penny pulls out her list of questions. She will say later that with each query, she is so busy thinking about the next one that she has trouble focusing on Lucy's answers. She asks about training for nurses, about what happens when a resident dies, about the evaluation her mom will receive to determine eligibility. She asks about the waiting list and how long her mom is likely to be on it.

This turns out to be a delicate question. "That depends on"—Lucy pauses—"turnover. It could be a year or two." After another moment of elliptical talk, finally Lucy says, "The only time I get a bed is when someone passes away."

"Oh!" Penny says, the idea settling in. "That's why you can't predict. It's not like going to a restaurant and waiting for a table!" She looks again at her notes.

She asks about the assisted-living facility next door, and whether her mother would be eligible to live there. "Your mother's

CPAP mask might be an issue," Lucy says. If Mary needed help with it, that would qualify as medical assistance, which the program does not provide.

The talk moves to Mary's financial situation. Lucy tells Penny that most of her facility's patients are on Medicaid.

Penny is surprised. Her mother is "nowhere near Medicaid," Penny says.

If Mary were "near Medicaid," she would be nearly poor. Medicaid is a public program that provides health insurance to low-income people. It is financed by both the federal and state governments. Coverage and eligibility vary from state to state. Massachusetts offers fairly broad Medicaid coverage to its residents, as part of the state's aim of universal health coverage. But a person older than sixty-five faces a strict assets cap: he or she must have no more than $2,000 in assets (not including one car, his or her home, and possessions) to qualify. Mary receives her small VA pension, Social Security payments, and, as a senior, is covered by another federal health-insurance program, Medicare. She will also soon inherit almost a quarter of a million dollars from her brother Gerald, who died last year. Penny will decide, with the help of expert advice, to have the inheritance transferred to an account held by her and her sister, out of which she will pay for any facility Mary goes to.

The inheritance is, in the most obvious sense, a financial boon: Mary's care will be paid for. Any institution she moves to will draw first from her VA pension and Social Security payments, and the balance will come out of her inheritance. Penny can continue working full-time, will not have to quit her job to ensure that Mary gets the care she needs. Many caregiving families would envy this scenario.

But the financial middle is, in certain ways and ironically, the worst place an ailing, elderly person can find herself in. A person with a little money, who is neither rich nor poor, and who lives long, often loses that money fast, as she spends it on expensive long-term care. Her assets will disqualify her from Medicaid—at first. She may end up "spending down" her money and qualifying. She will have to "make herself poor," in other words—just as a lawyer had helped William make Joan several years before—before qualifying for the program.

So develops an end-of-life conundrum for many middle-class people and their caregivers. Besides certain VA benefits, available to veterans and their spouses, Medicaid is the only national program that pays for many of the services and goods the very old typically need, such as extended nursing-home stays, "incontinence products," dementia day programs, and home health care. Medi*care,* the nation's insurance program for all elderly regardless of income and assets, doesn't cover these things, in part because it was created decades ago when people didn't live as long—when chronic illness among the aging wasn't as much of a concern. Medicare was designed to pay for acute care: surgeon's bills, emergency-room visits after heart attacks and strokes, and short-term nursing-home care after surgery, for example.

"I think it's shocking that the only way many people can get the care they need is to become poor," says Carol Levine, director of the Families and Health Care Project at the United Hospital Fund of New York. Levine says she does not expect, however, that the current options for paying for long-term care will change much in coming years. And she expects that the financial burdens of long-term care on families will increase.

At this nursing home, the Alzheimer's unit costs a staggering $9,000 a month, out of pocket. Medicare won't pay for it. But if a person qualifies financially, Medicaid will, although it will not reimburse the facility fully. In a nearby building, assisted living, with no medical care, costs much less—$2,000 to $3,000 a month, depending on services. With her inheritance, Mary could afford such a monthly fee—for several years, anyway. Depending on how long she lives, she may end up qualifying for Medicaid.

The biggest problem people face in saving for retirement, experts joke, is that they live too long.

Penny says to Lucy, "I can't let my mom go yet. I'd probably have to have a whole lot more meltdowns."

"Most of the people I see in this room," Lucy says, "are overwhelmed. You don't seem overwhelmed."

"You didn't see me on Saturday." Penny looks over at Inga.

Lucy takes Penny on a quick tour through the dementia unit. In a common area, Penny gazes at people in various degrees of lostness. One man sits with his head tipped back, mouth agape.

In the corner, a fish tank gurgles.

In the car, Penny and Inga conduct the postmortem. "I was looking at every face in there to see if they had that lost expression my mom gets," Penny says, heading the car toward the highway. "They're *more* lost. All those white-hairs—they could be my mom. But not." She glances at Inga, sitting in the passenger seat with her folder of assessment forms. "They're more like statues than human beings. It would be nice if you knew what was going on. If we knew *anything* was going on. They're at a whole different level of being than you and I are. Are they on the other side half the time? Or is this some purgatory they're in?"

"I don't think so," Inga says, referring to purgatory. "The brain is incredibly protective. When my mother had Alzheimer's, her brain protected her"—emotionally—"from her disabilities and her losses." In the early stages of her disease, Inga's mother was upset by her declining abilities. "She had the angry, I-know-what's-happening form of Alzheimer's." Inga's mother used to rap her head with her knuckles and say in frustration, "Not working." She loved to knit, and then she couldn't any longer. "But after the loss of being able to knit," Inga says to Penny, "the other losses were much less painful." With each loss of ability came an increasing loss of awareness—so that, Inga says, "incontinence, being in a wheelchair, needing assistance for dressing," seemed to cause Inga's mother less emotional suffering than these disabilities did Inga and her siblings.

The brain may be "protective" of the self in other ways, too. It wants to solve problems, achieve order. It fabricates stories, for instance, to explain confusing experiences. Early- and mid-stage dementia patients confabulate, make up stories, in an effort to explain—to themselves as much as anyone else—something they don't remember or understand. Sarah, for example, once said to her husband, "Honey, you left the car window down all night."

Without skipping a beat he replied, "I don't understand how that happened. Every time I get out of the car, I tap each window to make sure it's closed." Sarah knows he does no such thing, but she didn't correct him. He wasn't lying; he was making sense out of his own confusion.

Penny may be wondering, too, what sort of awareness those "statues" do experience. Has someone who looks completely "lost" also lost all awareness? Does he know, at all, that he knows—or know that he doesn't know? Does he know that he exists? Perhaps his mental state is similar to what we experience when we space out on a familiar commute: The mental experience of the drive consists of strings of thought, images, impressions, emotions—but no real *knowing* of this mental activity. We arrive home having forgotten the entire trip. Knowing that one knows seems to fade gradually with dementia, and to varying degrees. Liz's husband sometimes says, semilucidly, "Physically I'm fine. It's my brain. It's not quite right—yet." And then he goes on being confused.

In a support-group meeting, Rufus asks Ben, Can people with dementia *accept* their condition?

Ben pauses. "It's tricky. Because [acceptance can happen] on two different planes. You need the cognitive ability to process the construct of *acceptance*. Cognitively, you can't accept. You don't have the construct. But then there's the emotional acceptance, the 'I'm at peace with this.'" That, Ben says, seems more possible.

"The emotional, spiritual acceptance," Rufus says, nodding.

"It's complicated," Ben says. "There are a lot of things we still don't get about this. We're kind of walking in the dark."

Penny pulls her car into a second institutional driveway, past a sign that reads ALLEN MANOR, and below this, A CONTINUING CARE RETIREMENT COMMUNITY. It is the place near her house that she dropped in on a couple of months ago. She parks amid two-story, vinyl-sided boxes, arranged in a quadrangle. She has a few minutes before the next appointment. She and Inga fish out their assessment forms.

"'Good lighting?'" Penny reads.

"Oh, definitely," Inga says.

Penny makes a check in the yes column. "Are we having fun yet?" It is not a question on the form. Penny is feeling drained. So is Inga. "I'm glad I didn't try to do three places. Two are enough." Penny exhales and leans her head back. "I tell you, Inga, your doing this for me makes me know I'll do it for someone else."

"For me?"

"Pick it out for you? I wouldn't want to do that!"

"You can come visit me," Inga says. "On a good day, I'll say, 'Hi, Penny.' On a bad day I'll say, 'Who are you?'"

. . .

Christine, the marketing director, tall and energetic, leads Penny into a tiny office and describes the options at this facility: the gradations of care range from none to complete. I imagine a multi-tiered hourglass, sand moving down through darker levels, from sunny one-room apartment, through curtained nursing-home bed, unto the grave. Penny gets stuck on the difference between "independent living with assistance" and "assisted living." The difference, Christine tells her, lies in the degree of help—there is more in assisted living, but certified medical care happens only in the nursing home.

Penny's mother's CPAP mask comes up again as an issue. No one will help your mother, Christine says, put it back on in the middle of the night if she is in independent living, even if she is signed up for "assistance." She could get *emergency* help in the middle of the night, but if she made too many such calls, she'd be placed in assisted living.

"My ideal, anyway," Penny says, "is that she'll die in her sleep at my house. This is all just in case."

Christine leads Penny down a hall, knocks on and opens the door to an apartment in independent living, a small studio with one room and a kitchenette. Jane sits quietly in a rocking chair. She has tight white curls all over her head. She smiles amiably as Penny peers around the room, its white matelassé bedspread made up neatly. On a wall, someone, a daughter perhaps, has hung a calendar with photos of children, likely grandchildren, sitting on a stone wall, holding Easter baskets.

Ruth has a bigger apartment, with two rooms. Someone has hung her paintings—her own oils—all over the walls: village snow scenes with horses and carriages, a seaside vista, children playing in the snow. They are skilled, precise, evocative. Ruth is hard of hearing, but sharp. Her window looks over the parking lot. Christine tells Penny that the residents tend to prefer living on this side of the building rather than on the side with views of grass and trees. They like to see the action, she says. Penny says, "My mom sits and watches the kids in our neighborhood play basketball."

In the building next door, assisted living, Gertrude has just celebrated her one-hundredth birthday. Fourteen bright balloons fill a corner of her room. Down the hall, a woman named Alice sits in an embroidered armchair. She has a beautiful face, with fine features and calm eyes. She gazes at Penny. A black baseball cap lies next to Alice on a side table. "I like your hat," Penny says. Alice smiles.

In the car on the way back to Penny's house, Inga says, "My mother tried to stay on the farm when Dad died. She was seventy-one." Two years later, Inga bought her mother a condominium in town. Inga's mother lived there for thirteen more years. Inga called her several times a week, visited a few times a year. Other condominium residents checked on her. "The first time I knew my mother had dementia," Inga says, "is when I took her to Norway. She had this fear of the strange showers. She kept making excuses not to shower." Eventually Inga arranged for her mother to move to assisted living.

Penny pulls up to her house. A few of the rocks she took from the college campus are arranged in a corner of the yard; others wait in a pile. Mary is inside, on her spot on the couch, watching *Oprah*. Penny had said earlier that she was afraid to tell Mary that she needed to take Inga and me back to our cars at the pub. She worried that Mary would question this coming and going, ask what Penny has been up to. But Mary doesn't. Penny checks in and tells Mary she will be home again soon.

Back in the car, Inga says, "You're not ready to let her go, but you *are* ready to get those applications in so you have options."

Penny doesn't respond directly. "Part of me wants to tell her just what we did. But I don't know how to start it. I've got this big denial thing going." She turns onto the road that leads over the mountain. "I just want to get her away from the mind-rot box. From *Oprah* and all of that. It hurts my heart that she's happy with so little in her life." Penny wants to talk to her mother and say exactly this, that it is painful to see how she spends her days.

"Just be careful about what sort of abstract thinking you expect from her in return," Inga says.

"Yeah. Is it manipulation if I start crying?" Penny lets out a wry laugh, but no tears.

❧ (Mis) Perceptions

Back in November 2009, old friends invited Liz's husband, Joe, on a hunting trip—not to hunt, just to go along.

Against Liz's expectations, Joe went looking for his guns. He approached the cabinet where he had kept his hunting gear and found the lock changed. He conquered the lock (he had been a locksmith, after all) and discovered that his guns were missing.

Liz was unaware of this until a Sunday morning. She was sitting on the couch in their small den, and Joe appeared in the doorway, scowling.

"Where are my guns?!" he demanded.

Liz startled. "I had to get rid of them, for your safety."

Joe railed. He told Liz she was sneaky, horrible, that he wanted a divorce. His eyes were rageful. *"You don't know what I could do to you,"* he growled.

Liz felt cornered, more frightened than she ever had before

with Joe. He was blocking the doorway. She sat on the couch, not daring to try to exit past him. She remembers thinking, "Am I even going to be able to get out of here?" Eventually Joe stormed down the hall to the bedroom at the back of the house.

Liz grabbed her pocketbook and keys and drove to her son's house. Her son and his family weren't home. Liz used her key. She had the phone number that Ben had given her, should Joe get violent. She sat for a half an hour before making the call. Once she did, events proceeded as she had learned they would: A social worker arrived at the house to speak with Liz. Liz told her the story. The social worker said, "I can tell you're frightened. I can hear it in your voice. I can see it in your face. We're going to have to file a section twelve"—Title XVII, Chapter 123, Section 12, of Massachusetts law: if a physician, psychologist, or other mental health professional, after examining a person, "has reason to believe that failure to hospitalize such person would create a likelihood of serious harm by reason of mental illness," the professional may "restrain, or authorize the restraint of, this person" and seek to hospitalize him or her.

The social worker told Liz that the police would go to Liz's house and "frisk your husband. They'll have to make sure he's not armed or dangerous. In the meantime they'll call in an ambulance. The ambulance will take him to the psychiatric ward at the hospital."

"Imagine doing that to your spouse," Liz says, shaking her head. Liz waited a while longer at her son's house. A police officer called. He told Liz that Joe had entered the ambulance peacefully. The officer had found a pocketknife on Joe and left it on the kitchen table. Soon "emergency services called me," Liz says. "They said, 'We'll meet you in the emergency room. You need to bring the health-care proxy and the durable power of attorney.'" She drove home, got the documents, and drove to the hospital. By this time, Joe had been admitted to Ben's unit on the fifth floor. Liz arrived, and she remembers Joe railing, "She stole my guns! How do you think I feel about that? How would you feel if somebody took something of yours?" Later, "he refused to see me," Liz says. "Or talk to me."

A few months earlier, Liz had applied for a spot—a "bed"— for Joe at the veterans home. Not long before the final incident at home with Joe, she had learned that a bed would soon be available. A week or so after Joe was admitted to the psychiatric ward, a staff member from the veterans facility came to the hospital to assess him. Joe, Liz recalls, was still hostile and volatile. Looking back, her impression is that doctors had not yet found the right medications to calm him. He stayed for three weeks on Ben's unit. A hospital administrator told Liz that Medicare would soon object to Joe's extended stay. Liz was relieved the next day when the veterans home called: a bed was available.

Meanwhile a friend, Andy, had visited Joe in the hospital. During their conversation, Joe had told Andy about another gun, one that Liz hadn't known about. It's a loaded pistol, Joe said. I keep it in the coat closet. Andy, in turn, told Liz about the gun. Liz asked him to come to her house and help her find it. The two of them dug through the closet, finally finding the gun in the pocket of a vest. Andy unloaded the ammunition and took it with him. Liz stood in the kitchen, holding the pistol. It was about five inches long, cool in her palm. She had never before held a gun. She carried it down the stairs to the basement and dropped it onto a shelf.

During the period of Joe's escalating hostility, culminating with his apparent threat—"You don't know what I could do to you"—Liz had faced a dilemma, two competing troubles, the sort that social-work students might discuss in graduate school. On the one hand,

Liz had been responsible for an increasingly confused, frustrated man. Joe's ongoing "catastrophic reactions," outbursts, and hostility are common in dementia patients, even those placid before their illnesses. A social worker, all things being equal, might have counseled Liz to try to work with Joe's behavior: Be gentle, validate his feelings, go along with his delusions, try to see the world from his perspective. Persevere, the social worker might have counseled, learn some new skills—your situation might improve.

On the other hand, for fifteen years Liz had felt increasingly frightened, psychologically diminished, by her husband's behavior. Few experts familiar with the progression of domestic abuse would counsel a threatened spouse to stick things out. I asked Nina Silverstein, a gerontologist at the University of Massachusetts Boston, to reflect on the dilemma. Silverstein believes it shows the urgent need for better support in communities for dementia caregivers generally. Liz might easily have learned about, sought out, and received, for example, more specific, expert counseling around her daily care for Joe and his dementia, and opportunities to problem-solve, given Liz's history of being verbally abused. She might have been encouraged to take Joe to day programs at the senior center so she could get rest herself. A physician or geriatric care manager might have assessed Joe's illness more regularly and made referrals to other helpful programs. Such interventions, Silverstein suggests, might have prevented the final, sudden event that landed Joe in a long, disorienting, perhaps traumatic stay on a psychiatric ward not designed for dementia patients.

Of course, some problems—with all their complex factors—are simply, in the end, intractable.

In the first six months after Joe left home, into the spring of 2010, Liz visits him regularly. She decides that five times a week is acceptable—not because she wants to go, but because it seems like a schedule that will keep her guilt in check. Before long, she thinks she can manage only four visits a week. The strong, medicinal smells of the veterans home exacerbate her headaches. The emotional stress of each encounter wears her out.

In group meetings, members soothe her. William says, "After a while, he won't even know if you've been there the day before. That's the way it is with Joan."

Rufus says, "All I can think is, 'Oh, Liz has some relief.'"

"It's relief," Liz says, "but—"

"I know. It's hard," an occasional group member says. "You have a husband and yet you don't." This does describe Liz's dilemma, but not quite as the woman imagines.

Many moments carry such irony. During a visit to the veterans home, Liz watches as a patient looks Joe up and down. The patient asks Joe, "Why are *you* here?" The patient seems to mean, *You look fine to me, Joe.*

"That's what *I'm* wondering," Joe says.

"He's got some medical problems," Liz says.

"Oh," the patient says. "Well, Joe, you better take care of her." He gestures toward Liz.

"Oh, yeah, I will," Joe says.

Despite her resentment, Liz knows that the move to the institution has been hard on Joe, too. "It's a big loss for him," she tells everyone. "He says, 'You don't know what it's like not to be able to go out to your car with you,'" to go home. He says, "It just gnaws at me all the time that this is where I'm spending the rest of my life."

Liz says, "It makes me feel guilty, and that I should be there more when I'm trying to be there less." Meanwhile he says nice things all the time. "You're so pretty, Liz. You look so nice today." He says to other veterans, "That's my gorgeous wife." In the coming year, Liz will find such remarks more and more difficult to bear.

Sometimes he follows Liz out to her car, stands, and watches as she gets in. Tears well in his eyes. He says, "I should be home looking after you." Liz shares this comment with the group and manages a small smile. Perhaps they think she is describing tragic circumstances: a well-meaning husband, incapable of giving care. It will be a long time before she lets the group know about Joe's verbal abuse *before* his dementia became apparent. In the meantime, she tells only her daughter—and later, me—what has gone on.

Occasionally, she hears a comment that relieves her guilt a little. The facility's social worker tells her, "You don't want to wait until they get physical." In other words, it is better you moved him while you were both still safe.

Liz still finds a disconnect, though, between her perceptions and the staff's. "He tells them, 'I'm fine,'" Liz says, and they seem to believe him. Liz learns that a nurse has written in her notes from a meeting with Liz and Joe that Joe has "a little dementia." Liz wonders to the group, "What happened to the Alzheimer's?" Liz credits Joe's amiable affect, in part, to the mood-altering medications he takes. She wants him to be on them, yet believes that if he were not, she might get more validation from staff. They would "see what he's really like."

The use of psychotropic drugs—often dangerous for the elderly—in nursing homes has been an issue for reformers, who talk about inappropriate "chemical restraints." Seroquel, for instance, has been found to increase the risk of death among dementia patients. At least one small nursing-home experiment showed the effectiveness of replacing pharmaceutical approaches with behavioral ones. The lucidity of all nursing-home residents in the study improved when they were taken off the drugs. The problem, however, according to the Centers for Medicare & Medicaid Services, is that many nursing facilities do not have "systematic plans" for nondrug approaches to behavior problems. Many are still giving residents drugs such as Depakote, a mood stabilizer, and Seroquel, an antipsychotic medication. Joe receives both of these at the veterans home.

Liz is not aware of the risks; she simply knows that Joe is placid and credits the drugs. One day she finds out that Joe's Depakote has been cut in half and the Seroquel eliminated—perhaps the facility's response to increased public and government attention to the problem. Liz simply fears she will bear the brunt of any agitation that emerges—that her visits will be, at the least, unpleasant or, at worst, dangerous if she is alone with him.

Her worst fears are never confirmed; Joe often gets cranky with her, but never dangerous. Through the spring, Liz musters reluctant altruism. She struggles with self-criticism. "I'm my own worst enemy," she says to the group. She worries about what she will say to staff at the veterans home about the declining frequency of her visits, to friends who ask about Joe.

"You're still going through the transition," Ben says. "Joe was mowing the lawn a year ago—the last time the grass was growing." Seasons coming around again "could trigger stuff," Ben says, "and also, practically speaking, you have to deal with new challenges."

"I do have someone lined up to mow," Liz says. "A really nice guy."

Inga says that if Liz weren't a worrier, "she wouldn't have someone lined up. I'm the same way: I'm nuts, but I get it done."

"I just get so tense when I'm doing it," Liz says.

"Ants," Ben says. Everyone looks at him blankly. "A-N-T's." Automatic negative thoughts. Also called cognitive distortions. They make no sense," Ben says, but they're common. The term is used in cognitive-behavioral therapy, a form of psychotherapy that, by challenging dismal thoughts about oneself and the world, helps alleviate depression and anxiety.

"You think I've got cognitive distortions?" Penny says in a tough-guy voice.

"Hey, I have a collection of them!" Rufus says. "I'm a connoisseur of distortions."

"I can't wait to use that at work," Penny says, narrowing her eyes. "'I think you're having a *cognitive distortion.*'"

Everyone laughs.

As the year progresses, Liz becomes a support-group veteran. Giving advice, rather than receiving it, brings a kind of solace. At a meeting in mid-May, the group discusses a challenging notion: accepting dementia patients' misperceptions, rather than correcting them. It is a difficult principle to uphold, especially with someone you have long known. Karen breaks her usual silence and asks Liz, "When your husband asks the same questions over and over, what do you do?"

"I just keep answering him," Liz says, "like it's the first time I've heard it."

Karen peers at Liz quizzically. "You don't say, 'You *said* that already'?"

"I used to. When he was living at home. But it didn't work."

Karen shakes her head in agreement. "No. It doesn't." Don is sitting next to her, apparently listening. He shows no reaction. He likely doesn't know that Karen is referring to him, doesn't *remember* that he asks the same questions over and over. Karen turns to Ben. "Is that the right way to handle it?"

"Yes," Ben says.

"Shouldn't you treat them like a normal person?"

Inga says, "It's a disease. They don't have control over it."

Ben nods. "An extreme example is an eighty- or ninety-year-old woman who says, 'I want my mommy! I want my mommy!' You don't say, 'Your mother died a long time ago.' You say, 'Your mommy left, but she'll be back.' Because it reassures her. A moment later, she'll forget."

Sarah recommends a book called *The Validation Breakthrough*. It helped change standard approaches to intractable delusion. "When a two-year-old gets on the phone and talks to an imaginary friend," Sarah says, "we go along with it. But when an eighty-year-old talks in ways that seem like fantasy, we try to talk them out of it." In her earlier years as a psychiatric nurse, Sarah says, she was encouraged to do "reality checks: We'd say, 'No, it's not Wednesday. It's Thursday.' But things have changed. I'm learning it myself."

Liz turns back to Karen. "It's not easy to keep saying, 'Oh, really? Oh, *really*?' I still catch myself saying, 'Joe, you just *said* that!'"

The caregivers try to practice two kinds of skillful dishonesty: not correcting misperceptions, and also actively *deceiving* when necessary, to maintain a care recipient's peace of mind.

William says he tells Joan "little white lies. Like today, Joan said, 'Where're you going?'

"I said, 'Oh, I'm going to the hospital.'

"She said, 'Why?'

"I just said, 'Because I'm going to the hospital. I'll be back soon.'" He would be back, of course, but not until the following day. William has learned that keeping Joan happy is more laudable than perfect truth.

A Perfect Birthday

A chocolate cake sits in a plastic case on the conference room table, next to two bottles of ginger ale and a stack of styrofoam cups. Ben passes a greeting card furtively to his left. Daniel is sitting on Ben's right. The front of the card has a picture of a white-haired Albert Einstein and the words "My Theory About Birthdays . . ." Inside, the card says, "Age is relative." Group members sign and pass it along. Ben clutches a long metal knife. "Getting this out of a locked psychiatric ward was not easy!" He wields the blade over frosting and slices into blue, curly words: "Happy Birthday Daniel."

"It's terribly nice." Daniel pauses. "I really can't eat it, at my age." Daniel has incipient diabetes.

"We should be singing!" Liz says.

"Yes," Ben says. Karen starts off, low, *"Haaappy biiiirthday to you."* Others join in on disparate pitches. By the middle of the song, everyone has arrived at some semblance of a key. Certainly the singing is heartfelt. All applaud. "Speech!" Karen says, and Inga sings, *"How old are you? How old are you?"*

"Sixty-five, right?" Ben says.

Daniel will be ninety in two days. He smiles, a bit wanly. "It's tremendously kind of you." His face looks sad, tired.

"It really is amazing, isn't it," Karen says from down the table, "that we live so long?"

Daniel nods. "Yes. Yes, it is."

Ben offers Daniel a tiny piece of cake. Daniel shakes his head and holds up a hand, looking regretful.

Eighty-eight-year-old Don speaks up: "Since I'm a youngster, *I* could have a piece." The group laughs.

"Let's start with you today, Daniel," Ben says as people dip plastic forks into frosting. "It sounds like it was a hard week."

119

"Very hard." Daniel takes a deep breath. "Leanne was admitted to the hospital. Here." He points toward the ceiling. "She fell. I pushed that emergency button again. The same policeman came. He called the medics. They took her by ambulance to the hospital. This was about six or six thirty in the morning. She had taken too much medication. She OD'd." He pauses. "I mean, she wasn't trying to kill herself. She got mixed up."

Daniel says he has felt renewed affection for Leanne, seeing her so vulnerable. The group casts about for ways to help them both. Sarah suggests getting a nurse to come in and manage Leanne's medications. Ben wonders aloud whether Daniel and Leanne would have an easier time in an assisted-living facility. Daniel just says, "Thank you for the suggestions." He pauses. "I'm not very resourceful or—practical." There's dismay in his face, vulnerability. He takes a tiny bite of cake.

Moments of loveliness arise: respectful listening, laughter bubbling up in the midst of suffering, acts of compassion, encouraging words. The others in this group can do little concrete for Daniel—certainly they cannot change his circumstances. Yet the presence of others is its own solace. To become known, amidst a diversity of generations, personalities, situations, can be comforting. Inga says, "There's so much that everybody understands that you don't even have to say." People simply tell stories, describe circumstances, listen. Hearing about advanced stages of dementia helps prepare those who are coping with earlier stages. Meeting once a week seems to foster intimacy; stories unfold continuously and often in detail. There also seems to be space for difference, individuality.

Miriam, who, since the death of her husband, returns to the group occasionally as "the caregiver of Miriam," often tells a story to newcomers: James had become severely impaired and could not stay home alone. Miriam started bringing him along to the support-group meetings. She would ask him to sit at a small table in the corner. She gave him paper and colored pens. He drew and, as Miriam would learn, listened to the group's conversations. After one meeting, James—this man whose mind and physical abilities were falling apart—said to Miriam, "They're very nice people. They have terrible problems at home."

The group always laughs at the statement's irony. It illustrates a trend: Many members tell me privately that they find the support group helpful in part because they see others' problems as worse than their own. They think, "I don't have it as bad as she does," or, "At least my mother is sweet with me," or, "I'm grateful his mind is okay." Not quite schadenfreude, there is solace in recognizing others' struggles. The equation doesn't quite compute, however: nearly everyone seems to think that others' problems are worse than his or her own.

While Leanne is in the hospital, Daniel listens to music. He can't play piano any longer. This is in large part because of arthritis. Leanne reminds him, though, that he stopped playing for another reason, too: during the time they lived in a condominium, ten years before, he hadn't wanted to bother the neighbors with his playing. Now they rent a ranch house across the river, overarched by trees. Daniel no longer owns a piano. His nephew has acquired Daniel's father's baby-grand Steinway. It resides in the nephew's house in California, and Daniel's grandnephew is learning to play. The boy is only eight, but Daniel hears from his brother that the child shows great promise.

Daniel wishes that he himself had chosen music as a career. He wishes he'd gotten his degree in musicology rather than German and had taught music history. Looking back, he sees that international events intersected his life so closely that he became forever shaped by them. In choosing German, he feels, he never got free: distant horrors stayed present in his life. He regrets that he chose to study what seemed right—perhaps even convenient—at the time, rather than what gave him joy.

Daniel had said to me, during our first conversation in the hospital hallway, that he and his brother were "lucky." He meant, in part, that his father was both unusually prescient about what was happening in Germany, and unusually willing to send his sons to America. Daniel's father had traveled to the United States, had played with the great violinist Mischa Elman at his Carnegie Hall debut in 1908, and later with the famous American violinist Maud Powell. Daniel was eleven when his mother died of cancer. "That is one of the traumas—*the* trauma—of my life," he says. It was 1931, three years before his departure for America.

He tells me much of this over tea and apple pie at the hospital coffee shop. He is nearly always soft-spoken. When he gets animated by a topic, his voice takes on a breathiness. He sits up straighter, leans in, gestures with his hands. I express amazement, say, or ask him to confirm something he has said, and he squeezes his eyes shut, nods slowly, and says, "Yeah."

"My father did a brave thing," Daniel says. In 1933, he learned of an American committee that was bringing German Jewish children to the United States and finding homes for them. Daniel's father registered Daniel and his brother with the committee.

"They found a home for us. A Jewish family. In Philadelphia."

"It was amazing foresight," I say.

"Yes, it was, on my father's part."

"It would have been so easy to be in denial."

"Yes, as many people were. Well, he had the experience of being in this country, so he was more cosmopolitan. He spoke some English. So America wasn't a strange country." Daniel pauses.

"But it was a leap for him. He was a widower—and to send his two children . . ." Daniel shakes his head, a sad amazement on his face.

He takes a bite of apple pie.

Daniel remembers that it took a year for the brothers' application to go through. Once it was approved, his father learned that his sons would need to leave in a week. Daniel remembers being taken to the Cuxhaven port on the North Sea and embarking on a ship. He says he wasn't afraid. His aunt had told them, "You're so lucky to get out of here."

"That was the feeling we had," he says—of good fortune. Daniel was fourteen, his brother, Ernest, eleven. Daniel got terribly seasick on the ship. Perhaps, he says, this was partly an emotional reaction to leaving. They traveled to Philadelphia, moved in with a couple whose children had grown. Daniel enrolled in Central High School. Four years later, he graduated first in his class, earning a full scholarship to the University of Pennsylvania.

He graduated in 1942. World War II had begun. He joined the US Army. He and Ernest trained together in Alabama, surrounded by more red mud than they could ever have imagined. "Even though I knew German," Daniel says, "they sent me—this is a typical army story—to Ohio State and enrolled me in an *Italian* program." Daniel chuckles. "Italian is a great language. I enjoyed studying it. But . . ."

By late 1943, he says, the army "finally got into my German. They sent me to an intelligence training camp"—Camp Ritchie in Maryland, where Daniel and other German-speaking Jews learned how to interrogate German prisoners of war. He practiced giving a prisoner the impression that he already knew everything possible about German strategy. He and the others studied maps, rankings, names.

He went first to England and later lived with his interrogation unit in Belgium and then Germany. He wore a US Army uniform and questioned soldiers from the regime he had escaped, in his native language. He was simply an enlisted man, so he also spent a fair amount of time filling out reports. The interrogations weren't especially fraught. He was looking for information about troop movements, morale among German soldiers. He amazed one German soldier by mentioning details about Berlin that Daniel remembered from his childhood. The soldier assumed Daniel was revealing army intelligence.

"This was the last year of the war," he reminds me. The German soldiers "were glad to be out of the war, and to be in American hands rather than Russian ones. So they talked. Mostly. And if one didn't, there were a hundred others who would. The only ones who were difficult were the officers. I didn't get to speak to them very often. But I was there during the Battle of the Bulge. I remember when they brought in German soldiers dressed as Americans. They were infiltrating our alliance. It was really something. They said they were out to get Eisenhower. To *kill* Eisenhower. It was very exciting. Very dramatic. I think they were executed." (They were.)

Daniel offers the group an update on Leanne, who is home from the hospital. She seems a little better, although she's also talking about feeling depressed again. She talked to her counselor, who is going to consult with her psychiatrist. She walks a little better because of the physical therapy. She is doing exercises, including the bicycle—he turns to Ben—"which you were so kind to give us. In the meantime," he says to the group, "my own health has become a problem." His cancer, the non-Hodgkin's lymphoma, is surging. "My only symptom is that I'm absolutely depleted. No energy. My oncologist said I should have chemotherapy. The thing I'm worried about are side effects. How bad they'll be. My doctor said that this drug—it doesn't cure the disease; it just slows it down. He hopes it will kill cancer cells and not do any other damage."

"Wow. That's a lot, Daniel," Ben says.

"I guess so. Leanne was very upset when she heard this."

Ben nods. "That's a kind of shadow that's been hanging over you for some time."

"Yeah. In a way, yeah."

"Sometimes we dance around the question of what happens if you pass on. What happens to Leanne."

Daniel shakes his head. "Yeah. I don't know. At this point I really don't know. My work is essentially done." He gave a lecture recently on Nazi history, published an article. "The only thing that isn't done," he says, "is my work for Leanne."

The conversation circles around Daniel's cancer and chemotherapy. As Ben talks, Daniel has been turning to look at him periodically. Ben finishes.

Daniel nods. His face brightens a bit. "Would you permit me to tell a joke that is relevant to this situation?"

"Of course!" Ben says.

Daniel leans and hovers his fingers over the table. "A Protestant and a Catholic and a Jew have been told by their doctor that they're suffering from incurable cancer. They don't have much longer to live. So they get together to discuss what to do next." Daniel pauses.

"The Catholic and Jew ask the Protestant, 'What are you going to do?'

"The Protestant says, 'I'm going to see my minister, discuss the salvation of my immortal soul, and get ready for the next life.'

"And the other two say, 'That's fine.'"

Daniel nods and takes a breath. "The Protestant and Jew ask the Catholic, 'What are *you* going to do?'

"The Catholic says, 'I'm going to see my priest, confess my sins, and get ready to meet my fate.'"

Daniel nods again, signaling acceptance of the Catholic's intentions.

"The others ask the Jew, 'What are you going to do?'"

Daniel pauses.

"The Jew says, 'I'm going to see another doctor.'"

Daniel's eyes twinkle, and the group laughs.

His most radiant memory, he will tell me and the support group several times, is of May 8, 1945, after he'd been in Europe for about a year and a half.

V-E Day. Daniel's birthday.

He turned twenty-five in the little German town of Bad Hersfeld, four hundred kilometers from his birthplace, Berlin, on the day that the Allies accepted the surrender of the Nazi forces and secured the end of the war in Europe and of the Third Reich. "It was the greatest day of my life. To stand there in central Germany, in an American uniform, as a member of the Allied Forces!"

The day was clear and warm. Daniel climbed into a jeep with a fellow enlisted man, who drove—Daniel hadn't learned how—down the deserted autobahn (and across the line that would later divide East and West Germany). They pulled into Eisenach, the village of red-tile-roofed houses where J. S. Bach was born. Daniel's friend was a big fan of Bach's (Daniel less so), and the two men visited Bach's birthplace, a long, timber-framed house, "which had been damaged but not destroyed," Daniel says. From there they drove and climbed into the countryside to sprawling Wartburg Castle. "That's where Luther translated the Bible. Way up on this hill," Daniel says. "There was only a caretaker there, who showed us around. This huge place. There was *nobody* there. It was a *beautiful* day. We had a view of the mountains all over the place."

Daniel and his friend drove back to Bad Hersfeld, and that

evening, the members of their small unit, about twenty officers and enlisted men, had a party. Daniel got drunk for the first time in his life.

"I was making fun of the officers," he says, smiling, "which I had never done."

"You must have had such a feeling of release," I say.

"Yeah! Tremendous. After that long war. Yeah."

"They say the greatest pleasure is relief."

"Yeah. A tremendous day." He pauses, looks at me, then down, smiles slightly. He looks at me again, his eyes twinkling. "And they kept pouring. This was *hard* liquor."

"So at some point you don't remember any more," I say, smiling back.

"I only remember I had a terrible hangover the next day. But I remember that the more the officers poured into my glass, the more I made fun of them, and the more they laughed. It was a *tremendous* experience."

Daniel tells everyone that he wonders how he'll occupy himself during the chemotherapy and transfusion sessions. Each will take five hours. He says that a friend gave him an iPod, but he doesn't know how to use it.

Penny suggests finding a twelve-year-old to teach him.

Ben says, "You going to bring your Ozzy Osbourne tapes?"

Daniel looks at Ben blankly.

"Sorry." Ben waves the joke away.

"What about Leanne, when you're gone?" Karen asks from a few seats away.

"When I'm gone?" Daniel pauses. "Oh, during the chemotherapy. She'll be fine."

The hour is coming to an end. Ben says, "Thank you for being so honest with us, Daniel. I like what Penny says: 'You have to take it one day at a time.'"

Penny says, "You've been doing one day at a time for a while."

"Yeah," Daniel says. "At my age, that's all you can do."

People gather their things. Daniel leans forward and says, "I want to thank all of you for your friendship and support. It's been an interesting life."

"It's not over!" Penny says.

"Well, I'm very grateful to all of you. I'm happy that you've become my friends."

Sarah walks around the table, leans, and gives Daniel, still seated, a kiss on the cheek. Daniel receives it quietly. He nods and closes his eyes. He pushes himself up and stands. Penny approaches, wraps her arms around him, and holds him, rocking a little, back and forth. Penny appears strong—all that digging and hauling rocks—and Daniel looks thin, fragile, in her arms.

Memorial Day

One clear, warm morning in late spring, Liz watches over her grandson, Liam, while his parents work. She babysits Liam every Monday; the job is her source of joy. With Liam, Liz is a different person. Her anger, burden, regret, fade into a deep, if still muted, happiness. Caring for the little person nourishes her, even as she literally feeds *him*. The care is aimed, she says, at a happy future. She is helping someone through the upswing of life's curve.

In a small dining room, Liam sits in a high chair: blond hair, twinkly blue eyes, chubby cheeks. When he smiles, his eyes crease and become little downturned crescents. Liz sits opposite and keeps up constant baby banter. "Eat your blueberries, Liam. Who's a good boy? That's a good boy. Take the spoon! Who's the cutest baby? *Liam's* the cutest baby. What's the monster say?"

"Aaarh," Liam says, and grins at his grandma. He throws a couple of pieces of corn on the floor and smirks. "That's not funny, Liam," Liz says, suppressing a smile.

Pulling yogurt out of the refrigerator in the kitchen, Liz says, "Strawberry-banana. Yum." She reads the label aloud. "Yo! Baby!"

She moves a spoonful toward Liam's mouth. He grabs the spoon and sucks at the yogurt on it. He gazes coolly at his grandmother, shoves the spoon out to his side, and lets go. The utensil clatters to the floor. He peers down and smirks again.

"Not funny," Liz chirps. "Okay, all done." She holds her palms out to her sides. "All done. Can you do that?"

Liam spreads his chubby arms out. "Duh."

"Yes!" Liz says.

Out in the backyard, Liam walks stiff-legged and swaying, as if on high seas, across the grass. Holding his hands, Liz helps him up and down a plastic slide. "Wheee!" she says, and he swoops down, grinning.

She still misses Kevin, her first husband, the grandfather Liam will never know. Most of the time, she doesn't allow herself to think much about him. "He was a good man," she says. He'd grown up poor, one of the oldest among eight children. He became a helpful father, also comfortable with babies and children. They lived on a quiet, residential street not far from where Liz lives now. He died in a car accident late one night, on his way home from work. Liz was thirty, her twins eight, and older son ten.

The morning after the accident, sitting at the kitchen table, she said to her parents and the friends who had gathered, "Now I have to get a job."

But first Liz found herself hurrying, picking out a casket, making funeral arrangements. Eventually she did get a job, working as an aide to a disabled student at her children's school. In the months and years that followed, she found other, better-paying jobs and coped. She was living in a forget-and-move-on ethos—before therapy and bereavement groups were the norm, at least in her world; before they were as accessible and acceptable as they are now. "We didn't talk about him a lot in the following years," she says. Her older son had the hardest time. "Why did my daddy have to die?" he asked Liz many times. Liz found it impossible truly to console him. Looking for help, she called the priest of the Catholic church her family had attended. "Please come talk to my kids," she said.

The priest never showed up. Liz says, "That's when I stopped going to church."

She tells the group that the previous Monday had been the thirtieth anniversary of Kevin's death. "It was 'woe is me' over the weekend." She spent a lot of time in her house, in pain, alone with her thoughts. "It was, 'Everything happens to me, why does everything happen to me? Am I really a bad person?'"

"The ANTs were crawling all over you," Ben says.

"I go to a very dark place."

"Yeah," Ben says. "Have you ever tried meditation tapes or anything?"

"Yeah," Liz says without enthusiasm. "They help a little bit with a low-grade headache, but with a full-blown headache, nothing makes a difference."

"You suffer."

"I start thinking about Kevin," Liz says, "and about how he's never going to see his grandson."

. . .

Every Memorial Day, Liz visits Kevin's grave.

She drives Liam across town to the wide cemetery, its grave markers lined up, row after orderly row, where Kevin is buried. She parks, takes Liam's hand, and they walk under blue skies across the grass. At a flat stone set into the earth, she kneels.

Liam toddles among the other gravestones. Liz places her hand on gray rock. The sun is bright, the gravestone warm. Liam trundles over and joins Liz. He crouches, too. He flattens his palm and fingers and places his hand next to Liz's.

Liz gasps and smiles. The gesture moves her. "Liam," she says, looking down at him, "you have no idea what you just did." He turns and gazes up at his grandmother, his blue eyes squinting in the sun.

Later, Liz says to the group, "I hope I'll tell Liam the story someday. When he's much older."

"Put it in your journal," Inga says, "so you don't forget."

PART III

SUMMER

"Never Forget"

❧ Ambiguous Loss

For most of the caregivers, loss is incremental, a long vigil through steady decline. "This is *slow* grief," says a group member, Anne. "It just goes on and on and on." She has been caring for her eighty-five-year-old mother for years, through her mother's mouth cancer and radiation and liquid diets and chronic pain. "My mother is slowly losing everything. How can I not get pissed off?" We meet one afternoon in the hospital's coffee shop. Anne is fifty-nine, has chin-length, blond hair, and high, wide cheekbones. We sip tea. She says that for more than a decade she has nursed loved ones. Early on, she helped her mother care for an aunt with pancreatic cancer. Later she and her mother tended Anne's father, who had a rare, devastating brain disease. He gradually lost all bodily function, even as his mind remained lucid; he died in a nursing home about ten years ago. Anne watched over a demented aunt who lived in a long-term-care facility. Anne's husband has recently been diagnosed with rheumatoid arthritis and has heart problems.

"This whole caregiving thing, it's just unbelievable, the way my life has turned out with it," she says. "I get so angry, resentful at times." She had plans for her midlife years "that totally didn't happen. You never know what you're going to get. It's tough for people to understand," she says, unless they're going through it, too. Lately Anne has been consumed by the needs of her mother, who lives alone in a house not far from Anne's. Describing her mother's dependence, Anne tells the group, "She lives *through* me." Her mother has lost her sense of taste and has chronic pain. Doctors have been focusing on palliative care, on making her mother as comfortable as possible. Anne and a part-time home health aide prepare puréed foods for her mother, give her massages, and make sure she receives the latest medications doctors prescribe to try to ease the pain in her mouth.

Anne says she and her mother have always been close. This colors Anne's grief in a particular way: She grieves with great empathy for her mother and her suffering. "I'm living this *with* her," day after day. Meanwhile Anne has raised a daughter into adulthood and worked full-time in the hospital's administration. Responding to everyone's needs, finding time for some enjoyment, feels to Anne virtually impossible. She describes a marathon through slow loss. She remembers the same grueling decline with her father. She has talked in the group about envying those who lose their parents quickly. When parents go suddenly, she says, "you can grieve and move on."

Anne's grief is both protracted and unresolved. Pauline Boss, a researcher and psychotherapist, coined a term in the early 1970s to describe such loss and later wrote a book on it: *Ambiguous Loss: Learning to Live with Unresolved Grief.* A loved one is gone and yet not: "physically absent but psychologically near"—the abducted child, the soldier missing in action—or "physically present but psychologically absent"—beset by mental illness, enslaved by addiction, diminished by Alzheimer's. A long cancer or other cause of slow physical decline creates extended, stressful precariousness, too, just as dementia does. The strain of ambiguous loss,

Boss argues, exceeds any other. The uncertainty goes on and on; no rituals recognize it; no one can say when it will end.

The central challenge, Boss writes, is learning how to live with ambiguity.

Someone new to the group asks William, "Does your wife still know who you are?"

"Yes," William answers. "Just not by name."

Joan has been at the nursing home for more than four years. She is still around, but fading—and she won't get better. Apparently miraculous moments do come to pass: Joan, after not using her husband's name in years, asks an aide, "Where's William?" Another day she waves at William as he comes walking down the hall, with energy and clarity that startle him. Joan's bursts of lucidity are, over time, rarer, but they add to William's uncertainty. Dementia waxes and wanes.

William has gotten somewhat used to the surprises. One day as he is leaving her, Joan mutters, "Where're you going?"

"Home," he says.

"Well. I go there, too," she says.

William shakes his head, telling the story to the group. "And then it's gone." Another day "she whispered in my ear, 'You know I still love you?'" He smiles, rolls his eyes. "I'm thinking, 'Oh, here we go.'" Joan getting all lovey-dovey. Even now.

She says, "I'm ready to go home," and a moment later, "Where's home?" Perhaps she'd like to feel at home.

William's friend Roger visits Joan. She grabs Roger's hand. "She wouldn't let go for about a half an hour," William says. "She does the same with mine. She wants to relate to someone."

Ben nods.

William pauses, shrugs, and says to everyone, "I'm doing the best I can."

"You're doing great," Ben says.

"Like I tell Liz," William says, "you gotta keep your spirits up."

In May, William visits his place on Cape Cod. He gazes out at the view from his deck, watches birds riding swells on the shining Atlantic and whales breaching. "There are a lot of whales this time of year," he says to the group at the next meeting. "It was beautiful." When they bought the place back in 1956, he and Joan didn't know it would become valuable. Liz asks him about selling it. "Not yet," he says. "Too many memories there." The same goes for his house and workshop. Friends and family suggest he move to a condominium. William has looked at a few ads. But so far he isn't interested. Too many memories at home, too.

He struggles with the dilemma of artifacts. A few weeks after his trip to the Cape, William leads me on a tour of his and Joan's material history, through their small, bright kitchen, wood-paneled den, little living and dining rooms, up steep, narrow stairs and into the bedrooms, one on each side of a pink bathroom under the eaves. The house has hardly changed since he and his father-in-law built it sixty-two years before. In closets, on cabinet tops and shelves, he and Joan accumulated objects, more and less precious, over decades. In the den and living room, William placed wooden birds he'd carved—scarlet tanager with its black sleeves, bluebird, blackbird, cardinal, cedar waxwing with its bandit mask, wood duck, spotted plover, chickadee, titmouse, catbird, towhee, blue jay—on bookshelves and sills. In the dining room, Joan's collections crowd cabinets William built himself: hundreds of salt and pepper shakers, music boxes, and milk pitchers. "I go through twice a year," he says, "take them all out, dust them, wipe them down." Once a week, he walks around wielding a feather duster.

Our hopeful expectations of marriage include reciprocity, a symmetry of effort and affection. A relationship may fail as reciprocity does. Sometimes marriage survives obvious asymmetry. With aging and illness, with new dependence, if reciprocity flags involuntarily, the expectation of it can fall away—if relationships are to endure. William recognizes this. Two years earlier, he held a sixtieth-wedding-anniversary party for himself and Joan in her nursing home's dining room. Thirty people, mostly family, came. William recalls it in the support group: "The girls fixed Joan up real pretty. She still didn't know who anyone was. And she didn't know it was her wedding anniversary."

"But you've still got a marriage," Inga says.

William nods. "I've still got a marriage. Every day it's still a marriage."

William has stacked a basement closet with eight-millimeter films: *Cats,* Joan wrote once on one roll, and on others *my sister Hattie and her kids, California,* and *Grand Canyon*—her trips with William. On the other side of the room, on the walls above her desk, Joan once tacked newspaper clippings, funny photos of animals. They hang as before.

On the first floor, William pulls out a photo: he and Joan, in the early 1970s, wearing backpacks on Mt. Washington. "We camped right on the ground," he says. "We used to go with a dog, hike a ways, camp overnight. We tented all the way around Nova Scotia and Prince Edward Island."

He shows me a picture of their thirty-three-foot-long cabin cruiser, which he sold years ago.

"Do you call that a yacht?" I ask.

"I call it a *boat*!" He laughs. "We'd fish. Go over to Martha's Vineyard, Nantucket. It had everything—electricity, stove."

Upstairs in the bedrooms William points at Joan's quilts, her sewing supplies. He pulls out her wedding dress, yellowed from age. "It should have been in a box," William says, placing it back on a closet shelf. In the hall, a large cabinet holds some of Joan's old toiletries, nail files, and polish remover.

I ask, "Do you look at it all and feel overwhelmed?"

"Yeah. I think, 'What am I going to do with it all?'"

"Would you feel guilty if you just got rid of it?"

"Yes," he says. "Even now, if I give something away. One of my nephews visited with his little girl. She's about two years old. Joan had these teddy bears. I gave my niece one of them. I'd been holding on to it for four years."

"Everything's tucked away and tidy, though," I say.

"Yeah. I try to keep it that way. The way I was brought up—my mother had twelve kids, and that house was never a mess."

With his wife no longer able to keep doing her part, William takes on new roles and tasks. William tells one woman, new to the group, about his laundry folding, vacuuming, and dusting. The woman, about William's age, says, "Good for you!" and smiles. He chuckles. He has reason to be pleased with himself. Meanwhile, the woman is at home, doing the tasks her husband, wheelchair-ridden by a stroke, used to do. To her, it seems, they are hardly worth mentioning.

Women are still more likely to be primary caregivers than men are, but men are increasingly filling the role. Men's and women's care seem to show broad differences. Speaking generally, men's approach to caregiving tends to be task-oriented. They are more likely to handle finances and arrange for care from others, women to take on intimate daily tasks such as bathing and toileting. Men look for what needs fixing, problems that need solving. Women seek to nurture. These are overly broad generalizations, of course, but William does approach dilemmas with concreteness and practicality. Lately he has puzzled over this: Joan wheels around the nursing home, runs her chair into walls and doorways, and bruises a lot. The staff at the home can't figure out how to prevent her from hurting herself, short of restraining her. William considers the trouble for weeks. Eventually he and a few staff members figure out how to Styrofoam pipe-wrap the chair and protect Joan's limbs.

William meets Joan's needs as best he can. Then he seems able to let go. He frets over particular problems, but rarely stays burdened by guilt. In the group, someone asks him how often he feels sad. "You have to keep busy," he says. He feels low when home alone and idle, especially in the evening. But overall, he has achieved some peace of mind. He does what he can for Joan and every week gets together with Roger and Claudia and, several times a year, heads to the Cape, enjoys himself, putters, and makes repairs.

Meanwhile, for his devotion to Joan, he is admired by friends and the group. Women such as Penny, Sarah, and Liz, on the other hand, steeped since childhood in an *assumption* that they will nurture and give care, may receive less recognition. They may also acknowledge their own helpfulness less. As default caregivers, women's efforts seem more likely to be overlooked. Liz's guilty reluctance in her caregiving of Joe is compounded by social expectations she may barely realize.

Liz struggles with artifacts, too, but for other reasons. She cleans out Joe's pickup truck in preparation for selling it. She loads a few tools, road maps, odds and ends, in a box and stashes it in her—formerly his—garden shed. Not long after, Joe asks Liz for a map of New England. She says she'll bring him one. A few moments later he asks again. And at her next visit, he asks again.

She tells the group that she is not even sure she has one. She hasn't gone out yet to dig through the box from the truck. The map is probably at the bottom of everything.

Ben asks why Joe wants the map.

"He wants to show his buddy Jacob where he used to hunt in Vermont."

Well, that's nice, the group agrees.

Yeah, Liz says. But she's bothered. "You got a map of New England?" he asks yet again. She says, "No, not yet, Joe." To the group she says, "He doesn't realize that I don't just go home, watch TV, and eat bonbons!" Her headaches often disable her.

When one spouse no longer can, the other must. Sarah says on another day, "I think this is why I'm a witch, or what is it they say, a *bi-atch*? I'm realizing all the things that Walter used to do, that he's not doing now."

"Right." Ben nods.

At another meeting, Sarah says she recently got into her car and realized that the windshield-wiper fluid was out. Before this, the car needed an oil change. "All these things that Walter used to do. I'm starting to feel the loss in that. I'm trying to pick up the pieces all the time."

Another woman says, "I'm in that position, too. I have to go get the mail. I have to take in the trash. I have to put the barrels back in the garage. I have to change the lightbulbs. Each thing is easy, but, boy, it adds up."

Sarah nods. "Walter and I both worked a lot, but we had a wonderful partnership at home."

Ben says, "These little things have got to be done, *and* they represent an emotional loss."

"Yeah. The emotional loss." Sarah has to figure out how to do all the new tasks, she says, and also recognize that "Oh, yeah, now it's me that's doing it all." Divorced spouses often live the same dynamic—the new aloneness of domestic chores. Sarah will never have that old reciprocity back.

Around the outside of his house, William has planted petunias. Joan always loved this spring ritual, putting annuals into the ground. At the corner of the house, the exuberant, perennial peonies have finished blooming, their blossoms drooped and browning. "They don't last," William says. In his shop next door, he shows me the toys he has made from scraps of pine board—logging trucks, dump trucks, backhoes, tractors. He sells them, just for the enjoyment of it, out front by the road. He picks up a birdhouse and holds it out to me. "Take that. It's for chickadees. Hang it on a tree where there are bushes. They like to hide."

I make a fuss.

William shrugs and smiles. "I give three-quarters of my stuff away."

Back in the living room, I study photographs on the mantel: Joan with William's family in 1976, at his parents' fiftieth wedding anniversary, all the siblings lined up, the men wearing long-collared shirts. "That's my youngest brother. He died." He points at a sister: "She died." And another: "She died." He points twice more: "And both these two died." And then: "That's me. I was the oldest. I've only got four sisters left." He takes down a picture from his and Joan's fiftieth-wedding-anniversary party. "Joan had been tinting her hair. One time when we were in Florida, she was having a hard time figuring out the color. I said, 'Oh, just let it go natural.'"

She did. In her wedding photo from 1948, Joan has dark hair

and wears a white satin dress. I recognize her arcing brows; thin, long nose; and lovely large eyes. In keeping with her generation's rule against setting out personal photos, Joan never allowed William, throughout the decades they lived together in this house, to display the picture. Once she was gone—but still around—William took the portrait out and placed it on the mantel.

❧ Meltdown

One June evening, on her way to an AA meeting, Penny calls her sister Sophie. She needs to vent. She has had another conflict with their mother over walking. Just before leaving for the AA meeting, Penny had asked Mary to go out for a stroll. Mary had refused. Penny keeps hearing from doctors that Mary should walk at least once a day, and Penny takes this requirement seriously; she feels responsible. Yet often when she tries to get Mary to go out, Mary just settles deeper into the couch.

Describing their mother's life in Penny's house, Sophie likes to drawl, quoting the film *Avatar*: "She's dug in like a ti-ick!"

Penny tries to do the right thing, carry out the instructions of medical authority, but encounters real-world complications, messy human relationships and circumstances, and her best intentions get foiled. She finds herself powerless to fulfill this recommendation that is supposed to prolong and enhance her mother's life. Perceived failure can lead to guilt, which can lead to frustration, even rage. This evening on the phone with Sophie, Penny recalls a scene from their childhood: "Remember when our bedrooms were all upstairs? Remember I'd go around to you and Deb?"

Sure, Sophie says.

Penny would run to Sophie, who lay in bed, and say, *"I love my Soph!"* She'd kiss Sophie on the cheek. ("I was the baby," Penny reminds me.) Then Penny would scamper over to her other sister's bed. She'd say, *"I love my Debbie."* Another kiss.

This evening, on the phone with Sophie, Penny asks, "Well, you know what it is today?"

"What?"

"It's *'I hate my mother.'*" Penny weeps.

The next morning, a sunny, dry June day, I visit Penny at work. The college is out of session, the campus more quiet than usual. Penny sits at her computer, at a long, built-in desk against a wall of a small classroom. Across the room are school chairs with tablets, a whiteboard on the wall. On the door, Penny has affixed a nameplate she devised herself: PENNY JESSUP, O.C., L.M.S. The letters stand not for degrees, but for phrases her boss and a coworker, respectively, have used to describe her: "overcommunicator" and "Little Miss Sunshine."

She is still feeling stressed. A critical folder is missing from her database, she has just sent an urgent e-mail to a tech-support man, she's waiting to hear back—and meanwhile is still stewing about her mom. On her way to work, Penny called Inga to vent. She shares her meltdown with me, too. "I'm really upset." Every time she gets to this level of distress "is when I go and look at another place. For my mom. Have I filled out any applications yet? No. But I'm ready to look at another place *this week.*"

She is wearing jeans, low mules, and one of her flowered T-shirts. She checks her e-mails frequently and continues searching for the missing folder. Occasionally she turns back to me and talks about her mom again. The biggest frustration still is her mother's refusal to exercise. Penny often recalls Inga's advice to "get mad at the diagnosis" rather than at Mary. But "it's hard to get pissed at a diagnosis. It's much easier to get pissed at a person." After all, this supremely familiar person, her *mother,* refuses to walk. How could one's buttons not get pushed? One recent evening, she asked Mary to go out for exercise. It was raining, so Penny wasn't surprised when Mary said no. Later the sun came out. Again Penny suggested a walk. Mary again said no.

"I said to her, 'You know what? I do and do and do around here. I ask you to do this, and you can't.'"

Mary stays mum. "She knows I'm pissed and ready to argue," Penny says.

A pink plastic pig stands on the base of Penny's computer monitor, gazing smugly out at the room. A postcard on the cabinet above her work station says LIVE SIMPLY THAT OTHERS MAY SIMPLY LIVE.

"I feel like turning off the eff-ing TV. And saying, 'Mom, I'm sending you.'" Penny pauses. "I know that's not the way to do it. But that's how I feel."

Inga counsels Penny to try to keep in mind Mary's impairments. "She can't make a decision," Inga suggests.

Penny says, "She *did* make a decision. She doesn't want to walk!" Penny does try to remain cool in her caregiving, to be kind and not react—but sometimes frustration spills over.

Meanwhile Liz has been watching Joe's memory decline. She sits with him in the "canteen," a snack bar at the veterans home, eating the sandwich she has brought from home. Joe has already lunched in the dining hall reserved for patients. Liz finds it more and more difficult to come up with things to talk about. She asks Joe what he ate.

Joe thinks a moment. "It wasn't a hamburger." He considers for a moment longer and seems to decide: "Chicken and green beans."

"Oh. Did you have dessert?"

"No, just the spaghetti and one meatball," Joe says, apparently forgetting the chicken and green beans.

Conversations are turning ever more absurd. Liz takes note of the new and increased forgetfulness. She still feels, she says, that the staff "don't notice that his mind's getting worse." Liz is troubled, too, by Joe's declining social inhibitions. He often scratches between his legs as he sits with her in the lobby. The nervous tick makes him look, she thinks, as if he were fondling himself.

One day a big man walks through the building's front entrance. "Boy, that guy's fat!" Joe exclaims.

"Joe," Liz murmurs, "be careful what you say."

"*He* didn't hear me."

"Well, but what if he did?"

"I'm entitled to my *opinion*."

Telling the story, Liz imitates Joe's crabby tone. Another time, an aide walked by the doorway to Joe's room, wearing shorts. "Why would you wear those when you're so *fat*?" Joe said loudly, rhetorically, to Liz. Joe might have criticized people out of earshot in the past, Liz says. But the volume and apparent oblivion behind his remarks are new. Lack of inhibition is common in dementia patients, a result of damage to parts of the brain that control impulses. Joe can likely no longer reason through the impact of his comments nor prevent *thoughts* from coming out as *speech*. People with dementia sometimes behave inappropriately because they're confused and upset by their confusion. Liz knows that Joe's new behavior stems from his disease. (She also thinks it is possible he scratches himself because his medications make him itch.) Still, the impulsiveness is embarrassing, even frightening, to Liz. She remembers Joe's previous outbursts, threats.

· · ·

Lately Liz's headaches have been bad; she hasn't visited Joe in a week, she says to the support group. "I'm already feeling anxious about going back tomorrow."

"There's an objective for you," Ben says. "To get to the place where going does not make you anxious."

"Right," Liz says.

"Sounds like you're understanding some of the reasons why you *are* anxious," Ben says. "Like that staff might say, 'Okay, it's time to take him home now.' But also there's existential stuff: you guys are still going through a period of loss, the whole grieving process."

"Yeah. My therapist said it can take a long time, the acceptance."

"Absolutely. Years. You're getting used to being by yourself?"

"Yeah." Liz is living loss, sure, but she's also glad that Joe is out of the house. "There's no tension" now when she's home, she says. "I'm not walking on eggshells. There's some peace. I don't have to go in the bedroom and hide."

More and more, she says to me, she allows herself to think back on the way Joe treated her throughout their marriage. She realizes that Joe himself doesn't remember. "But I do," she says.

Few people know about Liz's burden of memory.

She is alone in general. Ben asks Liz, "Where are the people in your life who say, 'You're under so much pressure; let me take some things on for you?'"

"I don't know where those people are." Her best friend died of cancer a few years ago. Her children try to help, but they have busy lives, and Liz doesn't want to burden them.

Ben considers this an ANT, an automatic negative thought, a cognitive distortion. The group's conversation swings around, again, to the topic of negative thinking. Daniel offers his own, recent example: He had called an agency, needing to question a bill. He had steeled himself for conflict. "I was prepared for something dire to happen. But—nothing! They *agreed* with me." He chuckles.

Rufus says, "Ah, but if you hadn't expected the worst—I guarantee you, buttered bread always falls butter-side down."

Ben smiles. He suggests trying, in times of stress and negative thinking, "square breathing. It can be very calming." You breathe in four counts, hold four counts, breathe out four counts, hold four counts—and start over.

Penny listens. A beatific smile, perhaps ironic, appears on her face. She raises her eyebrows and clasps her hands in front of her sternum, as if feeling her diaphragm expand and contract. Her shoulders rise, pause, and lower.

"It changes the CO_2 balance," Rufus says, trying it briefly himself. "Of course, it doesn't take long changing the CO_2 balance before you pass out and die!" Rufus has his own, innovative automatic negative thoughts.

Everyone else seems to have his or her own version. At the next meeting, Daniel says of his latest troubles with Leanne, "She probably thinks I'm a lousy husband. But she doesn't say it."

Ben scribbles on a piece of paper and holds it up: ANTS. "That's an ANT, Daniel."

"It's also a cognitive distortion," Rufus says.

Penny giggles. "Are all ants actually cognitive distortions?" she asks, referring to the insect.

In mid-June I'm walking down the long, wide entrance lobby of the hospital on my way to a support-group meeting. I spy Daniel shuffling toward me, on his way out. We stop when our paths converge.

He smiles wanly, tips his hat. "Please tell everyone that I'm

going home. I just had a treatment"—a transfusion and chemotherapy for his cancer—"and I'm tired."

"Your first one?" I ask.

"Yes. It wasn't too bad."

"Did you read?" I'm thinking of the support group's asking
Daniel how he would occupy himself during the long treatment
session.

"Yes. I made some good progress on"—he leans toward me
conspiratorially—"*Pride and Prejudice.*" He'd told me weeks before
that he hoped finally to read it.

"I'm glad," I say, "and that it wasn't too bad."

Daniel is wearing his bomber jacket. It's a cool day. He tips his
hat again and steps toward the door.

🌿 Mary's Memory

In early July, I drive along the wide, flat river that flows south from
the college town to Penny's. It is time for Mary's annual memory
tests. Penny has invited me to come along. A neuropsychologist
will try to gauge deterioration in Mary's brain. The tests, for Penny,
hold a kind of power: they will measure, perhaps validate, her frustration and sense of loss. Caring for her mom is getting harder;
maybe the exams will explain why. Penny yearns for facts, evidence, understanding. More knowledge approximates more feelings of control.

When I arrive at Penny's house, she is standing in her garden,
watering the plants next to her driveway. Dressed in jeans and, as
usual, a flowered shirt, she sprays with a hose, peering through her
glasses. She points out new specimens to me: a tiny orchid; a big,
white, showy lily; cranberries in a tub buried in the ground. I don't
ask for the plants' Latin names; sometimes she volunteers them.

The beds hold a hodgepodge of flora, those of a collector, not a designer—showing as much interest in botany as beauty.

"We'll go in and see the mommy," Penny says, turning off the hose. Inside the gray ranch house, Mary sits in her spot on the couch, wearing a sweatshirt, the television running as usual. Mary looks up as I walk in.

"Mom, you remember Nell?"

"How are you?" Mary smiles warmly. I guess that Mary does not remember, but she doesn't let on.

"Mom, we have to go in fifteen minutes," Penny says.

"Okay." Mary hauls herself up from the couch. "I'm going to change my top. Is it cold out?" It's a cool day for July.

"You're going to want your jacket," Penny says. "We'll take your lavender one."

"Which lavender one?"

"This one." Penny takes it out of the closet by the door.

While mother and daughter change, the television plays a shopping program. Two women on the TV spend ten minutes extolling the attributes of variously hued thong sandals. "Bronze is really a *neutral* shade," one woman says. "You'll want to wear it with *everything*." Across the room, Penny's yellow orchids bloom, in pots by the picture window.

A plaque on a bookshelf reads IF NO ANSWER, LOOK IN THE GARDEN.

Mary leaves her bedroom, pushing her walker vigorously, listing to the left. She has a bad hip. Her shirt has black leopard spots and small purple flowers. She's put on white disk earrings. She looks almost polished.

"Where're we going? I can't remember," she asks. She's already queried Penny several times in the last hour. Mary shakes her head. "I can't remember *anything*."

• • •

In Penny's car, on the highway, with me in the backseat amid gardening supplies, Penny says to Mary, "This will be more than an hour of testing."

"Oh. It's a pain in the butt," Mary says. "What the hell are they checking?"

"Your memory."

"Oh, for heaven's sake. Who has a perfect memory?"

"That's a good point," Penny says, her eyes on the road.

"*Why* am I doing this?"

"Because of me! I started it. I'm causing all this."

Puffy, white clouds blow across the blue sky. I ask Mary if it feels good to get out of the house sometimes.

"Yes," Mary says, but this is perhaps an answer she thinks I want to hear.

Penny says, "I think you'd rather stay home all day every day."

"Yes. Oh, yes," Mary says, as if the idea is a relief.

"Especially if it's a doctor's appointment."

"Oh, yes!"

"They love you, though, Mom."

"That's because I don't bother anyone."

"Hah!" Penny guffaws.

"Except you," Mary says, as if dutifully.

"Yes. Except your daughter."

Penny parks by the entrance. She fetches the walker from the back of the car. She holds the walker as Mary hauls herself out. The three of us ride an elevator, emerge in a dull hallway, pass dull offices, open a door, and enter a windowless waiting room. Penny checks in with the receptionist.

Mary pushes her walker aside and eases herself into a padded chair. "It makes me sick. It makes me mad. I just got here and I'm mad already." She's frowning, but she doesn't seem all that angry. More like resigned, as if being angry takes too much energy. She blows out her cheeks, rolls her brown eyes, and leans her head back against the wall behind.

Soon Penny drops down between Mary and me, forcefully composed, clutching a five-page form. Mary looks ahead at nothing in particular. On the television in the corner of the room, Venus Williams lunges and swings at a tennis ball. Penny bends over the papers, including a three-page "Dementia Behavior Rating Scale." It asks the "informant"—Penny—to assess changes in her mother's slipping mind.

"I'll fill this out." Penny's layered bangs frame her face as she leans over. She's taken the day off to keep this appointment.

"Thank you," Mary says, leaning her head against the wall behind.

"It's nice to be appreciated," Penny says wryly.

"Oh, I do. I *do*!" Mary reaches up and strokes the back of Penny's head. "No one could have a better daughter!"

Penny purses her lips and scans the questions. She reads aloud the columns of responses: "improved," "no change," and "worse."

"I *haven't changed*!" Mary says, her brows knitting together, her face a near pout.

Penny turns to her mother. "You don't do crosswords anymore. You've started forgetting to take your memory meds."

Mary sighs. "I never feel old until I come here and you start filling out this stuff."

"Really, Mom?" Penny sets the form in her lap and turns to look at her mother. "What does it feel like to be old?"

Mary pauses. She gazes at a spot somewhere above the television, as if considering. "Kind of hazy." She grunts.

"Huh. Like hot and hazy?"

"No. *Cold* and hazy." Mary chuckles. Penny does, too, and turns back to the form.

There are a lot of questions. Trouble with cooking? Penny checks worse. Trouble with bladder control? A little worse, Penny writes in. Has drastically altered housekeeping habits? Penny quips, "Yeah, she's started *cleaning all the time.*"

Mary shakes her head.

Forgets to take medications?

"I *don't* forget to take my meds!"

"Mom, I wouldn't make it up." Penny adds, "Don't lay everything on me."

Mary just shakes her head again.

Penny finishes the form. The clinic's neuropsychologist, a small woman with short, gray hair, strides down the hall toward us and calls Mary. Another woman, behind the clinician, calls Penny. Penny and her mother traipse up the hall, Mary ahead, clutching her walker, her gait rocking and bent, Penny stepping along behind her. (Penny and Mary share the same sturdy build; one is simply more stooped and softened by time.) The neuropsychologist leads Mary through a door on the left. The other woman, dark-eyed with round cheeks, leads Penny and me into a room opposite.

Mary will spend the next several hours taking a "battery of specialized tests," according to a later report. She'll face down the Wechsler Adult Intelligence Scale, Fourth Edition (WAIS-IV); subtests of the Wechsler Memory Scale-Revised (WMS-R), the Boston Naming Test, the Controlled Oral Word Association Test (COWAT), the Token Test, the Shopping List Test, the Gollin Incomplete Pictures, the Right-Left Orientation Test, the Trailmaking A and B Tests, the Integrated Visual and Auditory Continuous Performance Test (IVA-CPT), the Verbal Absurdities subtest of the Stanford-Binet, Form L-M, the Mini-Mental State Exam, and the Geriatric Depression Scale.

She will draw clocks, try to identify objects by studying partial drawings of them, name as many words as she can that start with *F.* (Back in 2007, Penny documented in "The Golden Notebook" that Mary, for her first memory tests, recited, "friend, family, fun, fair, funiculi, funicula, fall, fare, fumes, full, and *flamboyant.*") She'll be shown a drawing of a boy and asked to put her left hand on the boy's right ear.

And so on. Inga will tell me later that *her* mother took similar tests way back in 1996. Inga says that Aricept had just come on the market, and to be prescribed it, her mother needed to be diagnosed with Alzheimer's. After taking the tests, Inga's mother was furious. She said to Inga, "No old person should *ever* be put through that!"

This summer, the neuropsychologist also asks Mary questions about her daily life. In response, Mary says that her memory has not changed since her last exam. She reports that she's had no medical problems. She doesn't think her medications have changed; anyway, her daughter organizes her pills for her. No, she doesn't drink, she says, and she no longer smokes. She has no problems with sleep, appetite, energy, or concentration on tasks.

She tells the clinician that she watches TV a lot. She likes it when no one bothers her. "After raising five children, I like having nothing to do."

Penny and I take seats with the round-cheeked woman in the office across the hall, which contains a mostly bare desk and three chairs. A single window looks out over a parking lot. Penny wants to know the woman's role. Is she a nurse? A social worker? "I have a bachelor's degree in psychology," she says. Her job is to ask the caregiver for information about the patient. She gazes at Penny and asks how things are going.

Few words are out of Penny's mouth before she melts into tears. "I'm getting tired of being the one to blame," she says, reaching for tissues. The moment, for instance, in the waiting room, when Mary insisted she doesn't forget to take her medications? "She doesn't *remember* that she doesn't remember to take her meds!" The woman nods. Penny goes on: She often gets awakened at night by her mother's going to the bathroom, by the "thunder" of Mary's walker in the hall. Penny can't get back to sleep, and she lies there, worrying: Will she, her mother's caregiver, the person responsible for Mary's life, know when it's time—when it will be necessary—for her mother to go to a nursing home? And what will happen then? How, for instance, will Penny's siblings react?

In two weeks, Penny will receive the results of the tests. Perhaps they'll relieve, a little, the uncertainty. Today she says to the woman in the office, "It's just really hard to watch someone lose everything they had."

At Last

Like Daniel, Inga has memories that younger people marvel at. She was born in 1939, but her childhood could be from a still-earlier time. She grew up in a wood-frame farmhouse "out on the windswept prairie of North Dakota," on her father's family farm, which they'd acquired under the Homestead Act. Until Inga was in high school, the house had no running water and no bathroom. The family used an outhouse. Inga remembers hauling water from a well in the backyard and washing dishes in a basin in the kitchen. She was the firstborn; her three siblings came along in the following sixteen years. Inga's paternal grandmother cooked for the household. Inga's mother made meals, too, and did housework and worked with Inga's father on the farm—out in the fields, and in the barns feeding chickens and hogs.

Inga was educated in a one-room schoolhouse on the prairie. In winter, the roads covered with snow—most of the school year, in other words—her father took her to class by horse and sled. In spring, when the roads were thick with mud, Inga had to skip school. Sometimes, the roads clear, her father took her and her siblings by automobile. Inga remembers that one day in her eighth year, she had been told that her father would be late in picking her up from school. She would need to wait for him. But Inga decided she didn't want to. She started home on foot, south on a long, straight road. Her house was three and a half miles away.

Before long, she spied a figure trailing alongside and slightly behind her in a field. A wolf. Inga slowed, and the wolf slowed. Inga hurried, and the wolf sped up. Inga kept on along the road; the wolf ran behind.

"My small heart beat, I tell you, so fast." Inga didn't want to turn back for school because she didn't want to be seen a coward. She kept watching that wolf out of the corner of her eye. Finally she reached a crossroads and turned west toward home. The wolf kept running south, away from Inga, toward the place where, Inga knew, a river flowed. The wolf had not been stalking her, she realized, just heading toward water. Maybe it was curious, too. She would never find out—nor walk home again.

Inga remembers her grandmother's strong hands, their large blue veins sticking up like ridges on a plain. The matriarch developed dementia late in life and continued living with Inga's parents until, in the latter stages of her disease, she moved to a nursing home. Inga had moved fast through school and graduated high school at the age of sixteen. She enrolled at the University of North Dakota. She wanted to study chemistry, but chose a field considered more suited to her gender: home economics. During college she met a local man who worked for a construction company. He asked her out. They married when Inga was nineteen. After she graduated from the university, she and her husband moved to a small Minnesota town, and Inga taught school.

Inga's daughter, Leisel, was born in 1965. Along the way, Inga's marriage fell apart, and Inga fell in love with a woman named Frances. In 1967, Inga and Frances ran away from the prairie with baby Leisel to New York City.

Inga and Louise met and fell in love in 1980. When Massachusetts authorized gay marriage in 2004, Inga didn't jump at the chance to make their relationship legal. Twenty-four years seemed like enough proof of their commitment. After Louise's return home from her final nursing-home stay in 2008, Inga and Louise simply practiced gratitude. "You know that stuff you see on the Internet?" Inga asks. "It's corny—but we *do* 'celebrate each day.' We say things like, 'Thank you for being alive.'" For months, Inga just tried "to go from emergency mode to not."

She says, "Now we're going to celebrate [Louise's survival] by getting married."

This July, they say their vows in a friend's garden, among a small group of guests, on a cool, misty day. A light rain starts in the morning and stops just long enough for the ceremony. "We wiped off the chairs," Inga tells the group the following week. A harpist played "At Last" and "Somewhere Over the Rainbow." The cake, too, proclaimed "At Last!"

Penny tells Inga that for most of her life, she has heard Mary talk about wanting to visit France. Mary could never afford to go. Now with her inheritance, Mary could manage the trip financially, yet her dementia and other health problems bar her from traveling.

Inga tells Penny, "We will bring Paris to Mary!" In mid-July, on Bastille Day, Inga and Louise show up at Penny's door bearing bulging canvas bags. They step into the living room, give kisses to Mary, who is embedded on the couch, and deposit supplies on the kitchen table.

"Are the croissants cut?" Inga asks. Penny has bought them, but forgotten to slice. She gets busy. Inga unloads a container of crepes she has made at home, and a dozen roses and small glass vases. She places flowers the color (almost) of the French flag— one red rose, one sprig of baby's breath, and one purple flower—in each vase.

"This," Inga says, holding up the purple bloom, "is what will pass for blue."

"*Trachelium,*" Penny tells me later. "A cut flower that nobody ever knows the name of." Inga places the flower arrangements on the kitchen table. She says archly, "I need *two* saucepans." Penny scurries to get them. Louise, meanwhile, has made herself comfortable in Mary's cushioned desk chair at the kitchen table. She lets Inga take charge. Penny turns the television off. Mary rests her head against the back of the couch and listens to the CD Inga has borrowed from the library: Édith Piaf singing "La Vie en Rose."

"I love this," Mary says, and closes her eyes.

Soon the women take their seats around the kitchen table. Inga serves cauliflower vichyssoise, croissants, quiche lorraine, fruit salad, and crepes with strawberries. "One crepe or two?" she asks as she serves, and adds strawberries and crème fraîche.

"I had only *read* about crème fraîche," Penny says later. "It's like sour cream on steroids, with sugar. Incredible."

Mary doesn't talk much during the meal. She does smile with enjoyment and compliments the food.

Penny says later that the brunch made her recognize anew

her mother's impairments. Mary seems unable to find meaning in such an event. "She appreciated it," Penny says. "But she's an in-the-moment kind of person now, you know? She had to be reminded and reminded and reminded the day before, and she had to be reminded after!"

Penny laughs.

At dinner that evening, after the brunch, Penny tells Mary that the leftovers they're eating came from that nice meal they'd had with Inga.

"Oh, yeah, that's right," Mary says, as if it had simply slipped her mind.

Penny receives the results of Mary's memory tests.

"Mrs. Jessup," the report explains, "primarily exhibited difficulties with short-term memory. She was unable to recall information following a delay regardless of modality or format (verbal list, story, or configural design). Her frontal lobe executive function skills, including planning, organizing, commonsense problem solving, and social sequencing, remained generally intact, although she had significant difficulty with logical analysis."

Later Penny's sister Sophie says she found the clinician's oral delivery of the test results, when they met with her, "a little belabored, a too-much-information kind of thing."

"Yeah," Penny says.

She, Sophie, Inga, and I are having lunch in a downtown café. "I didn't want the medical description," Penny says, eating salad. "I wanted the layperson's description." The neuropsychologist laid out "like, different kinds of *memory*, the frontal *lobe* stuff—"

"Don't *tell* me about the frontal lobe," Sophie says.

"Exactly. I don't want to hear about the frontal lobe," Penny says.

Penny reports on what was for her a remarkable family development. She'd e-mailed her siblings and told them the date and time of the meeting with Mary's neuropsychologist. Sophie had e-mailed back immediately and said she was coming. But Penny hadn't heard from anyone else. Penny and Sophie had driven to the meeting together. Mary stayed home. The sisters walked into the clinic's waiting room.

Their brother Steve—the sibling with whom Penny has had significant tension—was sitting in a chair. Penny felt stunned. He was the last person she expected to show up.

Here at lunch, the sisters talk about their surprise at his attendance and at some of the things he said. "Penny started talking about her emotions over having Mom placed in assisted living," Sophie says. Penny "got teary about it," the idea of moving Mary, about her desire to "just be a daughter" rather than a caregiver. Steve said, Well, when the time came to move their mother, *all* the siblings should let Mary know what was going on. They could *all* "explain what has to happen." Sophie turns to Penny. "*And* he said, 'We should all be there to help you when you do move her.'"

It was the sort of support Penny had been yearning for. Her fear of her siblings' reactions around Mary's care eased a bit, at least for now.

Returning to the topic of the test results, Sophie says, "Basically, Dr. Milton sees Mom as stable. But her memory issues are a little more pronounced." The clinician offered advice. "She said Mom does what we all go to yoga and meditation for—Mom lives in the moment. She's not five seconds *ago*; she's not five seconds *ahead*. If Penny can honor that, not criticize her for not remembering something, that would be good." Sophie takes a bite of salmon. "That's hard to do."

Inga says she thinks it's excellent advice. But, she agrees, it takes effort, mindfulness, to follow the advice consistently.

The clinician, Sophie says, counseled keeping every exchange with Mary upbeat, cheerful. That is the most important thing.

Penny nods. "The context doesn't matter," Penny says, remembering. "It's more important that both of you have a smile when you're finished. She was basically saying, 'Learn to accept.'"

Later, Penny will say to me, "Sometimes I look at my mom and I think, 'Not having any memory is kind of cool.'" Maybe memory loss partly accounts for why Mary is a "little Buddha." The neuropsychologist seems to agree, at least in Mary's case. But the notion that all dementia patients are lucky and live "in the moment" seems at the least simplistic and could, at the worst, deny patients' humanity and real suffering. But by advising that Penny try to be upbeat, the clinician is echoing what many other dementia experts say: calm, emotionally positive exchanges and experiences help keep people with dementia happy.

Tanglewood

Our selves depend on memory. Our experience appears seamless, our selves constant, because through memory our minds knit each moment to the next—from past, through present, and into the future. The past exists only as memory, the future only as an anticipation in our minds. Our relationships, too—with spouses, parents, children, siblings—are glued by memory. To put it in stark terms, a relationship exists because a person remembers who the other is, recognizes him. Joan does still remember William: she knows him, feels comfortable with him, seems to feel jealous if his attention strays. William remembers Joan with far greater intricacy than this—he carries stories of her in his mind, knows her old preferences, deeds, mannerisms, quirks. He structures his life in part to maintain these memories—pulling out Joan's milk pitchers and salt and pepper shakers, dusting them. He visits her every day in order never to forget.

Penny remembers her mother, the woman Mary was before. Penny's mind holds impressions of Mary, anecdotes, the sound of her mother's voice, the sight of her face when younger, ideas about her, both pleasant and less so.

Sometimes memory fuels division: misdeeds curse a relationship. If only we *could* forget. Liz remembers Joe and recalls fear.

Memories are plastic, often inaccurate, and always incomplete. Our memory of an event evolves, degrades, and differs from someone else's of the same event. We'll not remember every event nor every detail of the ones we do recall. James McGaugh, eminent brain researcher, has spent much of his career studying why we remember some autobiographical events more than others. We remember best, he writes, events to which we respond with great emotion. This is not surprising. McGaugh explains the phenomenon through brain science. It makes sense intuitively, too: emotionally charged events make more lasting impressions on our minds.

"Mahler," Daniel had said to me earlier in the summer, "is my favorite composer. I find him fascinating." We were chatting in the hospital parking lot after a support-group meeting. In July, Daniel said, Mahler's 150th birthday would come. At Tanglewood, where the Boston Symphony Orchestra holds its summer concerts—one of Daniel's favorite places—the orchestra would perform three Mahler symphonies, "including the Third, which is my favorite—for personal reasons." Into it, Mahler wove folk songs that Daniel grew up with. Daniel remembers marching to the tunes in ceremonies at his

German school. What Daniel loves about Mahler, however, is the opposite of nostalgia. He admires Mahler's irony, the way the composer "denationalizes" the tunes.

"They're no longer just German," he said that day in the parking lot. They "aren't patriotic or nationalistic; they're *existential*." He uttered this last word with reverence, gesturing with his right hand, long fingers spread, a graceful chopping motion. Universality moves him. He told me that, before he was allowed to serve in Germany in World War II, the army had asked him and his brother "to sign a statement, saying that we had no moral reservations about fighting our home country. We both signed easily." Daniel identifies with Mahler, another "man without a country." Mahler lived in the Austrian Empire and spoke German, but "was Jewish, not German. He had no nationality. I think that's why I'm drawn to him. I see myself that way, too."

We had inched our way across the parking lot. Daniel halted, spoke, walked a few steps with his cane, thought of something else he wanted to say, stopped again. He loves the post horn in the symphony's third movement, and the fanfare at the beginning. He looks forward to hearing the post horn played at Tanglewood, in the open-air hall. He thinks it will be *tremendous*. He plans to go to the Saturday-morning rehearsal. He has driven to these rehearsals every summer for decades. This year I'll go with him.

Leanne doesn't much like classical music—although, through concerts with Daniel, she has come to appreciate Mahler a bit. She likes rock, folk-rock, pop—music that Daniel abhors. Daniel tells the group that one recent day, he witnessed anew the cultural divide between them. Leanne had arranged for a cab to take them to an appointment at a hospital two hours away. Leanne sat in the front with the thirty-year-old driver. "They tuned right in to each other," Daniel says. They talked about rock music. Daniel sat in the backseat, listening, a little bewildered. "They knew all these performers. Leanne said, 'I saw the Stones and the Beatles and the Who.'"

Daniel pauses, shakes his head. "And she's married to this geezer."

"Aaw," the group protests.

"It's true!"

"ANTs!" Penny and Liz exclaim.

A little later, pulling his frail body upright, sudden defiance on his thin face, Daniel says, "I'll tell you something: In this country, you've got to be an optimist. You've got to be a sports fan. And you've got to be a capitalist. I'm *none* of those." Perhaps he believes that if he were, his marriage would be easier.

After serving in the army, in 1947 Daniel spotted an ad in the *Philadelphia Evening Bulletin.* The US government was requesting translators for Nazi war-crimes trials. He traveled to Washington, applied, was hired. He arrived in Nuremberg later that year. "I was assigned to a very nasty case, involving terrible atrocities"—the Einsatzgruppen trials. "These were the death squads in Russia that killed thousands and thousands of Jews, Gypsies, and other people the Nazis called 'useless eaters.' It was horrible."

Later on, the horrors would live vividly in Daniel's mind. But at Nuremberg, the content of the trials registered only superficially. He had to focus completely on the taxing work of live translation. "The grammar of German is very complicated," he says. "English is more linear"—generally, verb follows subject. In German, the syntax varies more. "This was so difficult. You had to guess ahead to what the verb would be." For this reason, "witnesses were told to speak in short sentences." Daniel sat in a glass booth with one other translator. Once a German defense lawyer "heard me say a verb before *he* had said a verb. He objected; he wanted it thrown out of the courtroom." Daniel says he pressed a button, illuminating a red bulb that signaled for the proceedings to stop. "I had to explain to the judge that I had to come up with a verb before it had been spoken."

The German lawyers were wary, Daniel explains. "The Germans knew there were a lot of Allied sympathizers, and a lot of Jews working for the prosecution. They suspected we would falsify. But we didn't. We were as accurate as we could be.

"It was the most concentrated work I've ever done. At the time, I was just doing the work. The content didn't register. I was concentrating on syntax."

"You were like a machine," I say.

"Yes. Years later, I gradually woke up" to the horrors. "The content came to the fore." Had he "woken up" sooner, Daniel says, he would have made different choices, would have taught music instead of German. But "I was already advanced in my field by the time I woke up," became fully conscious of, responded emotionally to, what he had experienced. He can't say exactly how the shift happened. It wasn't in graduate school, he says. His professors, while excellent scholars, were nationalistic, likely even Nazi sympathizers—although "they were careful" not to give themselves away. Perhaps studying under these men kept Daniel's emotions in check. Like many who grew up in Germany when he did, Daniel had an obedient personality. He was deferential toward authority—his father, teachers, professors—subject, ironically, to the same cultural forces that contributed to Hitler's rise. His "awakening," he says, likely occurred in the late 1950s and into the 1960s, after he'd left graduate school and begun teaching. In each of his language courses, he started spending an hour each semester teaching about Nuremberg and the Einsatzgruppen genocides. This helped further awaken him. Some of his learned compliance began to fall away.

"Nuremberg made me very anti-German," he says. Teaching about Nuremberg, even more so. Neither sports fan, capitalist, nor optimist, he is still, to his mind, not truly American, either.

Daniel finds out that the chemotherapy and blood transfusions have been successful. The progression of his cancer has slowed again. He will carry on through an old age made possible by modern medicine. In fact, Daniel's primary-care physician tells Daniel he will likely die of something else. He feels he has been granted a reprieve, a great release from fear.

In mid-July, in the early cool of what will grow to be a bright, hot day, I meet him, according to his instructions, before seven, in a parking lot by the river. We drive, I at the wheel. At seven forty-five we roll, wheels crunching, onto the quiet and nearly vacant Tanglewood grounds. We enter a ritual that Daniel and other devotees have observed for decades: the procurement of good seats for a Tanglewood Saturday rehearsal. Only one woman, Nadine, has arrived before us. "Hello, Daniel," she says. Daniel takes a seat in a folding chair that he has brought along. By eight, six people stand behind us; Daniel knows many of them. He nods and smiles. He introduces a few to me as friends. One man, an ebullient professor of engineering, greets Daniel with a hug. A woman tells me brightly that she has been coming every summer Saturday, but "only" for nineteen years. She is seventy-one, a violin teacher in New Jersey.

The line grows longer. Only one or two people look younger than sixty. Accents are redolent of Long Island and New York City as news travels along the line: So-and-so has cancer. Another is in hospice. One couple is missing for unknown reasons. The sun rises higher and the air warms. A gate attendant steps down the line and rips our tickets in advance so that, once the gate opens, we'll be free to dash for seats. A signal squawks over a walkie-talkie, and the gatekeeper motions for us to pass. Nadine jogs ahead of me across the impeccable lawn, past thick and sprawling oaks, toward the enormous Koussevitzky Shed. I follow, into the vaulted space. I pick a couple of seats close to the stage, in the center. Others file in behind. A woman calls to me, "Daniel would want to be farther over! So you can get a good view of the conductor!" I move toward the right. The good seats are filling up. A small woman to my left, silver hair in a bun, calls, "No, he would want to be over here!"

I see Daniel with his cane, making his way into the shed. "I don't know where to sit," I say, smiling.

"This is fine." He nods toward the stage. We take our seats just to the left of the podium.

There is more waiting, and a talk by a musicologist. Eventually members of the Tanglewood Music Center Orchestra wander casually onto the stage. They sit, tune their instruments, chat. They're young—teens and young adults, musicians-in-training, and already among the most advanced musicians in the world. The conductor, Michael Tilson Thomas, strides on, makes a few remarks comparing Mahler's enormous piece to a national park. The symphony is the longest in the "standard repertoire," three hours. Tilson Thomas will today take the orchestra through only parts of it.

A symphony, Mahler said, should "contain the whole world." The Third is his ode to the natural realm. It is so sprawling and dynamic that at times it sounds unhinged, full of dissonances and extremes in melody, dynamics, instrumentation. Two percussionists run left and off the stage and play a distant, unseen solo. A moment later they hurry back on. Daniel listens, rapt. The symphony is in part a hymn to summer. Outside, the weather and grounds comply: Green lawns glisten; the sky is nearly cloudless; the air has grown hot. Soft breezes move through the Shed and cool us. In the third movement, Daniel's gnarled hands rest in his lap. He raises one finger and points to the left. He nods in that direction, solemnly—he's anticipating the post horn that reminds him of his childhood, but broadens its meaning. He takes a great breath inward. The horn sounds, offstage, as if way up a valley—sustained, sweet, elegiac—a song of leave-taking.

Daniel wipes a tear. He will say later that hearing the horn is, for him, like "a distant reminiscence."

At the end of the last movement, the audience applauds heartily. Tilson Thomas waggles his hand, an "it was okay" motion to the timpani. Daniel says he thinks the young people played wonderfully. "Mahler is so vivid. Each instrument, each part, just jumps out at you." And the post horn, he says, "is haunting."

On the way home, he speaks more of living between worlds. He loves many things about this country, including what he sees as its openness and inclusive values. But he has spent most of his life not fully inhabiting it. He seems to me a tragic romantic—who loves a fiery composer without a nation, who yearns for other eras, the old country's food, seemingly for a place he cannot name. The past "haunts me more now than then," he says. "I would never have gone into German had I known."

He regrets his choice not just because he realized an aversion to German culture, but because the subject tied him to his past. For solace, every week in summer for more than forty years, he has traveled to hear music that transports him. Today, I drop Daniel off in the parking lot where we started. He drives home toward domesticity and, although he would never call it such, his quiet heroism, his caring for Leanne.

🌿 Guns, Cars, and Sex

In late summer, Sarah has a piercing dream: She is working as a nurse, "taking care of everybody"—doing what comes naturally to her. A vague and disturbing presence skirts her awareness: A person hangs from "some sort of wire or rope. He was dangling, just dangling!" she says later. In the dream, even though she is busy caring for others, she can't ignore the man on the wire. She takes a moment to assess the others. She says to them, "You're all right. I have to go over *there*." She heads to the person hanging on the wire.

It is her husband, Walter. She reaches with her weak arm—the one injured by a former psychiatric patient—and tries to help him. She wants to save him. But she's powerless. She cries, saying, "Walter, I don't know what to do! All the people here are sick. I don't know who to call for help."

Later she thinks about the dream: She was good at her job as a nurse, felt competent, helpful. In her marriage now, caring for Walter, she feels inadequate. She blames Alzheimer's, this confusing disease, for her impotence. Sometimes, she says, she wishes Walter had cancer. She would know what to do.

Dependence, and caregiving, no matter the disease, bring shifts in roles and relationships. A parent who once gave must now receive. A spouse who always navigated now gets lost. A caregiving spouse who always deferred to greater skill or assertiveness must now take charge.

Sarah tells the group that she fears that Stop & Shop is going to fire Walter. His balance is poor; he has a hard time concentrating on tasks. A manager recently called and left Sarah a message, asking her to come in and chat. Sarah fears that the manager will say that Walter has become a liability. But Walter loves working, Sarah reminds everyone. She worries that if he loses his job, he'll give up on life. "Throughout our marriage, he has said that if anything happened to him, he would kill himself. I believe that he could. That's been a mantra of his, that he's not going to be a burden, he's not going to bring me down, he's going to want me to move on with my life."

She pauses. "So the guns have reared their ugly heads."

She reminds the group that Walter was a cop. "He has several guns from his work. Three-seven—what do you call them? Seven forty-sevens? No, that's a plane." She laughs.

"He could have a thirty-eight special, or a three fifty-seven Magnum," Rufus says.

"Right. He has three fifty-sevens," Sarah says.

"Or a Glock nine."

"He has a Glock," she says, nodding.

"Yeah, they all have Glocks," Rufus says, referring to cops. "What you can do, if you're not going to do anything about the guns, is secure the ammunition."

The ammunition is still at home, Sarah says. "We moved the box of guns, my girlfriend and I—it's extremely heavy—into my closet. He never walks into my closet."

"Is the three fifty-seven a revolver or a semiautomatic?" Rufus asks.

Sarah pauses. "I don't know. It's silver with a black handle."

"Does it have a cylinder?"

"It has a cylinder."

"Okay, that's a real gun." Rufus demonstrates how to remove the ammunition: "You push the lever on the side, the cylinder comes down—*phhth!*—out come the shells. You put them in a bag. You take the Glock—there's a button on the side, the clip comes down."

"They're shell-less and clipless."

"Good! That alone is a big insurance policy. Ammunition is really easy to deal with. You know anybody who's still a shooter?"

Yes, Sarah says, but he is a long drive from here.

"Can you bring it to the police station?"

Sarah rejects the idea of bringing the ammunition to the station where Walter used to work. She wants to deal with the guns anonymously. Maybe she'll bring the ammunition up north to a station in a town where Walter isn't known—

"They *will* make a report," Rufus says.

"That's what I was afraid of." Sarah pauses, shrugging. "Maybe," she says half seriously, "I'll just throw it all over the bridge into the river."

"No, no, no," Rufus says. "Someone sees you do it and the next thing you know, you're suspect number one."

In general, experts say, dementia caregivers should try to remove objects that "cue" dangerous behavior. Jackets hung on door-side hooks might cue walking outside, which could lead to getting lost. The gun cabinet in Liz's house may have cued Joe to look for his guns. Car keys—and cars—cue driving.

In addition to guns, the group often discusses another danger: impaired driving. For Karen and Don, it is a persistently contentious issue. Don has always driven the two of them. He still does. Karen sits in the passenger seat, alarmed by his confusion. She speaks up about the issue for the first time at a meeting that Ben cannot attend. A few people have gathered anyway. The conversation comes around to Don and Karen's struggles. Rufus tries acting as dementia marriage counselor.

Don sits quietly, wearing a light-blue cardigan and a US Air

Force cap. Rufus turns and speaks in Don's direction. "Don's really doing fine—"

"Ask Don if he can drive downtown," Karen interjects.

"Of course I can," Don says, sitting straight, his blue eyes blinking behind wide glasses.

"I know you can operate the automobile," Rufus says. He leans forward, gesturing with his fingers toward Don. "What're your odds of getting back home?"

Don says firmly, "One hundred percent." He shakes his head. "This is not the right part of the conversation."

"You may indeed be capable of doing so." Rufus seems to be sidestepping. "But"—he turns to Karen—"it would worry you sick, wouldn't it?"

"Oh, absolutely." Karen crosses her arms.

Because dementia increasingly impairs driving and creates risk, people with dementia will at some point need to stop driving. But judging a person's driving competence is fraught with power dynamics. Karen and Don are in the thick of these, and Karen's frustration shows. One late-summer afternoon, Karen and I cross the hall to get water in the cafeteria. "My problem is anger," she says—meaning Don's anger, not her own. "He gets enraged. I think he doesn't want to believe this is happening to him. I get furious when he gets angry. I don't know what to do." She describes Don's forgetfulness, his repetitions. "It's like dealing with a *child*. I'll be honest with you. I fell head over heels in love with the guy. He was so dynamic, funny, competent." She pauses. An implied *but* hangs in the air. "This isn't the man I married."

In the group, she listens to Sarah talk of love and grief; she sees Sarah cry. "Where does the love *come* from?" Karen asks, here in the cafeteria. She seems to mean, How do I love someone who, in my eyes, is no longer lovable? "I admit sometimes I think about divorcing him. He says it, too, sometimes—that he's going to leave."

. . .

It's true: Sarah does still love Walter, deeply. Her love has changed, though, in distressing ways.

In our conversations outside the group in coming months, Sarah will talk with me about what seems to her a taboo subject: sex in a caregiving relationship. She never hears people mention it. For many years, she says, she and Walter had a fulfilling and romantic sex life. They'd married in middle age, never had kids together. They traveled a lot and enjoyed making love in creative places. But as Walter has become more impaired, the intimacy has shifted. Physical troubles have arisen; Walter is in pain and not as, well, vital as before. But a more important, and heartbreaking, shift has occurred in Sarah's mind: Walter's dependence on her alters everything. She gets him ready for bed at night; she rubs lotion onto his feet; she helps him in the bathroom. "If he has an accident, which he periodically has," she cleans him. She washes his clothes, removes stains. "I'm somebody else now." She feels more like a mother than a lover. Sexual intimacy doesn't seem appropriate. "This is like, *incestuous*," she finds herself thinking when Walter's touch becomes charged, erotic.

In months to come, the question of sex will arise less and less. Her relationship will move, inexorably, beyond it. The following year, Walter will move to a nursing home, the same one Joan lives in. He will go there for rehab after surgery, will fall repeatedly, and his cognition will rapidly decline. Sarah will decide that he needs to stay. Sometimes she will imagine climbing into bed with him there, just to be held. She'll mention this need to the aides, and they will say, Sure. Just please pull the curtain around the bed.

Walter will express his love for her in new ways. Before, he only rarely said, "I love you." But he would reassure her, "You can tell how much I love you by the things that I do for you."

During this time, Sarah will say to him, "I know you love me."

He will say, astonishing Sarah, "But now I'm not *doing* anything for you. Now I want to *tell* you." He'll say, "I love you to the moon. I love you to Pluto. I love you to Mars."

At a summer meeting in 2010, Ben talks about the grief of changing relationships. "When Penny's mom was younger," he says, "she juggled the responsibilities of a large family." Mary, he knows, was capable, vital, funny, curious. He turns to Penny. "But you don't see that very much anymore. You probably miss it." Penny nods. Ben turns to Don and Karen. "Sometimes, for a person who's going through changes, you have a vision of yourself—you have a vision of the other person—as the manager of a fleet of bombers, of a summer camp. But now, things are different."

"That's right," Karen says. "That's what happens." Her face softens into sadness for the first time ever in a meeting.

"It's hard. It's hard," Ben says, nodding. "It's about grieving the life that we had."

Hitting the Brick Wall

Late summer is exceptionally hot and dry. Tree leaves curl and crisp, flowers shrivel, lawns turn brown. At a mid-August meeting, a newcomer, Claire, shows up. She is forty-eight, a divorced single mother, tall and slender, with shoulder-length, dark hair. Five years before, Claire and her mother, Harriet, arranged to have a handicapped-accessible apartment built as an addition on Claire's home. Claire's father had vascular dementia and had gone into a nursing home eighteen months before. He had died while the apartment was being built. Claire's mother financed the addition, having sold her home, and moved into the apartment under a use-and-occupancy agreement; Claire continued to own the house, including the apartment.

The arrangement seemed like a smart way for Harriet to age "in place"—avoiding a facility—close to her daughter and grandchildren. Still, "people thought I was nuts," Claire says. For several years, all went well. Harriet watched the kids after school while Claire worked. Claire and her mother, who had always been close, continued to get along well. But beginning in 2009, Claire became increasingly troubled by her mother's behavior. One afternoon, Claire's daughter called Claire at work. The "house smells disgusting; it smells like stove," her daughter said. Harriet must have left an unlit burner on, but couldn't smell the gas leak. Perhaps most disturbing was Harriet's staunch denial that anything could be wrong. Claire called a neighbor, who walked over to the house, adjusted the stove's knob, and opened windows and doors.

Later, in the fall of 2009, Claire accompanied her thirteen-year-old son and his class on an overnight field trip to Martha's Vineyard. Crossing to the island on a ferry, Claire got a call from her ex-husband. He said that Harriet had called and told him that she couldn't care for their daughter that afternoon. Claire phoned her mother. Harriet reported that she had fallen the evening before, on their porch. She had taken some oxycodone and figured she'd wait to see if she felt better in the morning. She didn't feel better. She told Claire that her head had been bleeding and her neck hurt.

"I have some first-aid training," Claire says, "so I immediately recognized that she was talking about a head-and-neck injury." Claire hung up and called an ambulance. A few moments later, unable to reach her mother on the phone—the 911 dispatcher was keeping Harriet on the line—Claire asked a neighbor to check on Harriet. The neighbor reported seeing blood all over the porch.

"I freaked out," Claire says. The ferry docked. She, her son, and his classmates got on bikes and began pedaling to a youth hostel. A hospital physician called Claire while she was en route. "The good news," he said, "is that there was no brain damage." The bad news was that Harriet's neck was broken. He was sending Harriet to a bigger hospital farther south.

Claire left her son and his class, took a return ferry, and drove two hours to the hospital. She found Harriet on a gurney, in a neck brace, alone in the hallway of the hospital's emergency room, waiting to be seen.

Fortunately, the fracture in her vertebra hadn't severed her spinal cord. Harriet had surgery about ten days later. She went to a nursing home for rehab and then returned home. Right away, Claire noticed that her mother's mind had taken a turn for the worse. Harriet's and Claire's troubles escalated. Harriet forgot pots cooking on her stove next door; Claire smelled burning. Once Claire ran over and threw a smoking teakettle into the snow; another time, a pot of potatoes. The gas-leak problem recurred several times. Claire persuaded her mother to get an electric stove. Harriet became lost taking Claire's daughter to a violin lesson, and Claire persuaded Harriet to stop driving.

"It was challenging to set limits," Claire says. "But I did."

In the spring of 2010, Harriet fell again at home. A windstorm had blown through the night before. Fetching the morning paper, Claire found a tree blocking Harriet's front door. Claire used the interior door between her home and her mother's and found Harriet on the floor, near the bathroom, unable to get up. "She'd peed on herself," Claire says. Claire couldn't help her mother stand. "She couldn't bear weight."

Claire called an ambulance, again. The EMTs entered Harriet's apartment through Claire's house, which Claire found upsetting because her children had to witness the "drama."

The ambulance took Harriet to the hospital. Doctors found

that she had broken her pelvis. Harriet went to a nursing home, again, for rehab.

She is still there, Claire tells the group this day in August. Harriet's Medicare coverage has run out. She is demanding to return home. But the head nurse at the nursing home, and Harriet's physical therapist, both believe Harriet is not well enough to live alone. She has poor judgment and balance, they say. The year before, after Harriet had broken her neck, a physical therapist had urged Harriet to use a walker. But Harriet had rarely complied. Now the nurse and the therapist are exhorting her to use a wheelchair. They say that even using a walker, Harriet is likely to fall. Claire is certain her mother will refuse to use the wheelchair, as well.

For Claire to make decisions legally on her mother's behalf, against Harriet's own wishes, a psychiatrist must find Harriet incompetent—unable to make decisions for herself. Claire recently arranged for an assessment, but the psychiatrist found Harriet competent. "He believed everything my mother said," Claire tells the group. Therefore, Harriet's physician has told Claire, Harriet "has the right to go home and hurt herself."

"He told me," Claire says, "that he thought she *would*" hurt herself—"that it was inevitable," and no one could do anything.

An ombudswoman from a local elder-services organization moderated a meeting among Claire, Harriet, and Harriet's providers at the nursing home. The meeting went badly. "All relations broke down between my mom and me," Claire says. "My mom said some pretty nasty things to me. She'd always been critical of me—but this was a new level." Claire found the meeting so upsetting that she skipped the next one regarding Harriet's care. "I was devastated."

She tells the group, "I can't endorse a plan that will result in her getting splatted on the floor again." Claire, who says that her mind generally tends to spin toward worst-case scenarios, fears that her mother will cause a fire and jeopardize all of their lives. She fears that her mother will not just fall, but *die* in the apartment next door, and that she, Claire, will walk in and find her—or worse, one of the children will.

Months later, Claire will tell me that, during this time, she decided to remove herself from all decisions regarding her mother's care. She found the emotional cost of the dilemma too high; she had children and a full-time job to attend to. "I could not take responsibility for taking care of her." Claire says she could have refused to house her mother any longer, out of both a sense of principle—it didn't feel right to allow her mother to put herself in a dangerous situation—and self-protection—Claire feared for herself and her children. Legally, as sole owner of the house, she could have evicted Harriet from her home. Claire saw clearly that this was the worse of two unfortunate options: let her mother return home and face the risks, or evict Harriet and likely force her onto the state's elder-protective services.

The group listens, engrossed by the starkness of Claire's dilemma. "Her doctor told me," Claire says, looking around, "that I'm just going to have to separate myself emotionally." She grimaces, fighting tears. "You can see what a great job I'm doing!"

"Oh, it's the easiest thing in the world!" Rufus says.

"She's only my mother, after all."

The group nods sympathetically. Sarah asks Claire whether she gets support from other family members.

Claire shrugs. She has one brother. "He actually visited recently," she says wryly. "He stayed for about forty-five minutes!"

There are nods and murmurs of recognition: Claire is describing a familiar sibling dynamic.

Teary, Claire digs into her bag. "I can't believe you guys don't have a box of tissues."

Rufus pushes the napkin container across the table toward Claire.

"The napkins are thicker," Sarah says. "Trust me!"

The air-conditioning whirs; it's cold, as usual, in the conference room. No one can figure out how to turn the AC down. Liz has wrapped herself in a plush gray shawl. Karen wears a heavy cardigan.

"Note to self," Claire says, helping herself to a napkin and wiping her eyes. "Next time, bring tissues—and coat." She shivers, and laughs along with everyone else.

Claire says her mother has always been stubborn, but this quality has intensified since Claire's father died, and since her mother's health and circumstances have deteriorated. Tending to *difficult* loved ones intensifies the baseline emotional strain of caregiving. One's efforts to help, to keep safe, to soothe, are frustrated by maddening obstacles—erected, perhaps unintentionally, by the care recipient. The caregiver experiences the usual challenges of meeting demands in too little time, figuring out the various riddles of care—but the puzzles are compounded. She feels not just loss and anxiety about an uncertain future—but also hurt, frustration, and anger in reaction to another's lack of cooperation, even hostility.

Such challenges arise not just with difficult care recipients; sometimes the complications arise through unhelpful or difficult friends, neighbors, siblings, or other family. Sometimes it is a combination of several of these. Unresponsive siblings, insensitive family members, oblivious friends, *and* uncooperative care recipients are frequent topics of conversation in the support group. Months later, one member will say wryly that her sisters "always manage to be unhelpful in surprising new ways." Coping with difficult people is a common topic for empowerment sessions: the group urge one another to ask for help from people who are able to give it, to set limits on those who are chronically unhelpful, and to find ways to let go when possible and take care of themselves.

That August day, after describing her predicament to the group, Claire sits, composing herself.

Rufus leans over the table toward her. "May I ask you a personal question?"

"Sure."

"Have you hit the brick wall?"

A woman who's been attending for the last few weeks has heard Rufus mention the "brick wall" before and asks, "What is this wall you've been talking about?"

"It's something that happens to caregivers. It happened to me. It happened"—Rufus gestures up the table—"to Sarah." Sarah nods. "It happened to several others here."

Claire looks at the ceiling, fighting tears. "How do you know if you've hit it?"

"You just lose it. You hit a wall. You love a person, you want to *do* for the person. But your whole life is nothing but abject misery."

"I just want it all to go away," Claire says.

Rufus sits back. "You hit the brick wall."

"Mm-hmm," others murmur.

"We are the other side of the brick wall," Rufus says almost triumphantly. He likely doesn't mean that the support group will eliminate Claire's troubles and stress, but that empathy from the group, and information, can make situations—and one's reactions to them—more manageable.

"I actually hit [the wall] a couple of weeks ago," Claire says soberly. "I just couldn't get here." She couldn't find anyone to watch her children.

In late summer, Liz hits her own brick wall. Sitting with me one day on the plush brown couch in her living room, she says, "You caught me on a frustrating day." She is vexed by the staff at the veterans home, particularly the social worker, who has not been returning her calls. Joe's behavior, Liz feels, is getting much worse. She is ever more wary of visiting him. She and he don't have anything to talk about, he's getting hostile toward her again, and going there makes her headaches worse.

"I don't know how much longer I can keep this up."

"I get the sense you're feeling a lot of *anger*," I say, like a therapist.

"Yeah." Liz releases the word like steam.

The dedication of some of the group members amazes her, especially William's. He has reached an iconic status in the group for steady devotion. Liz also marvels at Sarah, and Inga. She wonders what they would think of her if she confessed that she doubts her commitment to Joe, to visiting him. She watches the other wives at the veterans facility arrive for their daily visits with their husbands.

With the loss of Kevin, her first husband, she says, "It was like, 'That's it. He's gone.'" With Joe, though, she can't know how his disease will play out: Will Joe end up "like the guys in the locked unit"—the Alzheimer's ward—at the veterans home? "They don't speak; you have to remind them to swallow; they lose control of their bladders and their bowels." She sighs. "I don't know how long I can keep going up there."

Illness—your own and someone else's—surprises, even shocks. Liz says, "You never know what's coming." Suddenly you are outside the gates of normal—your own sense of it, and the world's. Who knows how to respond, what to expect? This is not the script you've learned. This is not, you're certain, who you are.

Not long after I visited her at home, Liz falls seriously ill. For twenty-four hours she is bent by coughing and abdominal pain. Eventually, reluctantly, she calls 911. When the ambulance arrives, she's embarrassed by the state of her hair, her dumpy clothes. At the hospital, she has a CT scan of her abdomen, and despite no clear evidence of infection, doctors diagnose diverticulitis. They also suspect pneumonia. They administer ciprofloxacin. Liz reacts to the antibiotic. Her blood pressure drops dangerously, so low she can barely speak. She's wheeled to the intensive-care unit. Frightened, she thinks, "This is it. I'm going to be pushing daisies." Her lungs fill with fluid. For the next several days, she's in and out of consciousness. She'll remember being poked, prodded, intubated. To the specialists who see her, Liz is a riddle, a problem to be solved. A pulmonologist removes a liter of fluid from her lungs. For a trans-esophageal echocardiogram, Liz must swallow a tube— an "awful experience," she says later. A rheumatologist examines her, but reaches no conclusions of which Liz is aware. She remembers that "an infectious-disease guy" also took a look, but she never hears back about that exam.

She spends nine days in the hospital. During her time in the ICU, her son and daughter-in-law visit. They bring good news: the baby they're expecting is a girl; Liam will have a little sister. Liz cries with happiness. A nurse asks with concern, "What's going on?" Liz assures her that it is good news. Later Liz will say she thinks the nurse wanted to protect Liz, that the nurse suspected Liz's son was causing trouble about inheritances. "A lot of patients don't make it out of there, and people know it," Liz says.

I visit her in the hospital the day before she goes home. Standing in the doorway to her room, I see her lying flat in bed. It takes her a moment to focus on who I am. "Nell!" she says. She smiles wanly. Her auburn hair is tidy as always. Ben had visited her several days before. He'd said, "Hi, Liz. You taking visitors?" She'd said, holding her hands to her eyes, "Yeah, but you might not want to look at my face!" Today, with no makeup, following an ordeal, she does look tired, small, diminished—yet newly relaxed somehow, perhaps relieved, certainly less guarded.

She tells me hospital stories: A young doctor, perhaps a resident, put a central line into her chest. He had difficulty getting it in. He tried various places, finally pushed it into a spot just below her left clavicle. Later it was bleeding, looked awful. The clinician came back and said, "Why don't you look away."

She did. She heard a click that sounded like a camera. "What— you're taking pictures?"

"Yeah, for my Facebook page," he said drily.

"Of your ugliest patient."

She is on steroids and as a result has gained twenty pounds of fluid. This annoys her. Her daughter, Julie, will come today and bring her home. Liz hasn't seen Liam; he's not allowed in the hospital because he's too young. She misses him, can't wait to hold him.

Julie stays with Liz at her house for the next several days and, during one, brings Joe to visit. Joe sits with Liz, who dozes a lot on the couch. She fears he might say, "I want to go downstairs and see my tools," most of which Liz has gotten rid of. But Joe seems to have forgotten them, for the time being. He does say, "I should be here taking care of you." To her relief, though, he says this only a few times.

🌿 Twilight

One early-September evening, I drive to Penny's house for dinner. Just before I arrive, Penny will tell me later, she and Mary had an argument about going for a walk.

"Why don't you just leave me alone!" Mary cried.

"You always feel better after you walk," Penny said.

"Oh, *all right* then. Let's go now. Let's go *right* now."

"Are you going to pee first?"

"Oh, all right then." Mary shoved her walker down the hall.

I knock. Penny calls me in. Standing in the living room, I see Mary emerge from the bathroom, carrying a black cardigan. She spies me and smiles warmly.

"Hiii," she says serenely, the argument apparently forgotten.

"Oh, aren't you a *sweetheart*!" Penny says from the kitchen. She eyes the ceiling briefly, exasperated. "Mom, if you put on a sweater, you don't have to keep it on. It's warm out."

Mary stands by me in the living room, her arms aloft and in the sweater's sleeves, the rest of the garment draped over her head and face. "I'm getting aggravated here."

Penny walks over and tugs. Mary's visage appears.

"Are you going with us?" Mary asks, her brown eyes wide. She's speaking, apparently, to Penny, not me. "Because if you're going with us, we better get going." Perhaps Mary thinks I'm here to take her out myself.

"You talking to me?" Penny says, making a joke of the confusion.

"You talkin' to me, lady? Huh?" She smiles and puts her arm around her mother's shoulders. Penny goes to the door and opens it. Mary pushes her walker with force over the threshold.

"She's going to run me down!" Penny says.

"I have to push hard to get over that thing," Mary says.

Mary chugs up the block, stops, turns her walker, and sits, puffing. The three of us chat. Penny tells me she's been using a Havahart trap to catch red squirrels.

"You have a what? A heartthrob?" Mary says.

"Havahart trap," Penny says, laughing. "I haven't had a heart-throb in a while, Mom."

"Oy vey," says Mary, the Catholic. "I can't keep up with you, Penny."

"Anyway," Penny says. "I'm trying to get the red squirrels, but I'm not catching the little buggers. They're hiding black walnuts underneath my porch. I got a black walnut, drilled it, wired it inside the trap. Caught two of the squirrels finally."

"What'd you do with them?" I ask.

Penny whispers conspiratorially, "Sent them over the river," took them to a place from which they couldn't get back.

"*I'd* hit them over the head and throw them in the trash," Mary says.

"Mom, you can't hit them over the head when they're in a Havahart trap. How would you do that?"

"I don't care. I don't care." Mary frowns. "If you're going to use a trap, why not kill them?"

"Oh, you mean, like a giant rat trap."

"What's the point of catching them in the first place?"

"Just to *remove* them from my area. I think it's bad karma to kill them."

"Karma. What kind of karma?"

"The karma that follows me around."

"What do you think is going to happen to you?"

"It's what has *already* happened to me. I'm making up for bad karma."

"Oh." Mary shakes her head, looking a little grumpy, a little confused. "You're crazy."

"Yes, I am. And you're lucky that I am as crazy as I am."

Mary softens a little, grunts. "Yes, I am lucky."

Penny puts her hand on her mother's back.

"Oh. Scratch there," Mary says. "No, lower. Lower. *Lower.* Right across there."

"Right around the bra strap."

"*That's* what it is," Mary says, and closes her eyes.

After dinner, we stay sitting at the kitchen table by the window. Pictures of grandchildren are stuck to the fridge, a stack of bills and mail lie at the end of the table.

"Did you make coffee?" Mary asks.

"You said you'd be okay with water," Penny says.

"Yeah. I just asked."

"If you want me to, I can."

"No."

Mary says to me, "Well, if you've got any questions, ask me now. Because my program is on soon."

"Don't mess with *Jeopardy!* Or *Wheel of Fortune*," Penny says.

I ask Mary about sledding with her sister, a story I heard on the tape of memories she made.

Mary laughs. "I was heading right for the back stairs, and I hit my lip right on the corner. I still have a scar there." She shows me a small, white hyphen in the left corner of her mouth. "My sister said, 'Don't go down by yourself.' But I did. *That* was for not listening," she says, fingering the scar. "I still don't listen. I do what I want to."

Penny nods. "The walk, that's the only thing we argue about, usually. But she always feels better after she goes."

"Oh, I do. I know I do." Mary looks up at the clock. "My program's going to be on in about five minutes."

Mary is sitting on the couch. A contestant cries out, "Front. Page. News!"

"Yes!" says Pat Sajak.

Bells, whistles, cheers, contestants' shrieks, ring through the kitchen and living room. "Okay, you've got nine hundred dollars, what do you want to do?"

"I'd like to *solve,* Pat!"

"Okay!"

"Picture. Perfect. Performance!"

Penny stands by the kitchen table, leafing through "The Golden Notebook." She glances at the television. "It is what it is," she says drily.

"The sound track to your life," I say.

"Right."

Penny finds a pile of mail and emptied-out envelopes on the sideboard behind the couch. She holds out a mass mailing addressed to Mary Jessup. "Look, Mom." Penny reads aloud, "'The Gift That Lasts!'"

"I don't want that," Mary says from the couch, waving it away. "I don't read it." She keeps staring at the screen.

Underneath the pile of mail, Penny finds a brown bag with a slice of bread and a pat of butter inside, left over from Meals-On-Wheels, from who knows when.

"Call now!" the TV implores. "Or order online! One. Eight hundred. Pet-meds!"

Penny and I step outside. We wander around in the quiet twilight, looking at plants. Penny talks about her recovery work, and about trying to get Mary to walk, and about learning the difference between kindness and insisting on the truth.

Nearing the house again, I hear the TV, still busy. I think I hear an announcer intone, *"Seven thousand, seven seventy-seven, two thousand seven, GMC, three-quarter-ton pickup truck!"* It doesn't make sense, so I can't be sure it's what he said. The world is full of small confusions.

PART IV

FALL AND EARLY WINTER

The Far Shore

🌿 "A Good Death"

Months ago, back in March, because Mary's elder-care lawyer recommended it, Penny drove south to a funeral home in her Connecticut hometown to make arrangements for Mary's cremation and memorial service. Doing so, the lawyer said, would help "spend down" Mary's savings, should Mary need to qualify for Medicaid, and would relieve Penny and her siblings of this expense after Mary died. Before Penny's visit, the funeral director had sent Penny forms with questions to answer. Penny had found herself able only to glance at them. They were questions she preferred to avoid: Earth burial? Mausoleum entombment? Cremation? Viewing? Name of cemetery? Executor's name? Damn.

Sophie met Penny at the funeral home, and the sisters sat again with the questions. They chose "The Lord Is My Shepherd" as the prayer for the memorial service. They decided that a deacon from a Catholic church in town would preside over the service. Mary's body would lie in a sheet-lined corrugated-cardboard box and, according to Mary's wishes, would be cremated. Her ashes would go in the same wooden box that had held Penny's father's ashes. Penny and her siblings had since scattered his remains.

· · ·

If only decline and death were as amenable to plans, as straight-forward, as preparing for its aftermath. "Life is pleasant. Death is peaceful," Isaac Asimov wrote in one of his novels. "It's the transition that's troublesome." Diagnosis, decline, suffering, the final days—they're difficult, even grueling; dying is hard work, say those who tend to those going through it. "We rarely go gentle into that good night," writes the physician Sherwin Nuland in his seminal book, *How We Die: Reflections on Life's Final Chapter.* If we knew the work of death and faced it and prepared for it—and gave help through the process with courage and wisdom and skill—perhaps the passage would be easier. So while a caregiver's intentions are to ward off harm, to advocate for needs, to extend or enhance life, keeping death in mind as the inevitable outcome of elder care-giving, even if years away, may make for better decisions—may make for a kinder, easier time. "This is going to end in death," Penny had exclaimed back in February. Caregivers' main intentions rarely include consciously escorting someone toward death. Still, one hopes for as gentle an end as possible, and the privilege of helping make it so.

This fall, Claire—the divorced mother who'd come to the group in late summer and talked about her mom, Harriet, who had lived in an apartment in Claire's house, broken her pelvis, gone to a nursing home, and then insisted on coming home against Claire's wishes—continues fretting over Harriet's care. Claire returns to the support group only once after that first time in August. In September, she starts a new, full-time job teaching school, and the group's meetings conflict with her schedule. I catch up with her later, over phone conversations, and once in a downtown café, and learn about the whole "troublesome transition," as it unfolds for Harriet.

Not long after Claire's visit to the support group, friends from Harriet's church find Harriet a home health aide, a woman who works independently, and Harriet moves back into her apartment in Claire's house. The aide, Susan, helps Harriet a few hours each day.

Claire had feared calamity should her mother return home, but in the following months no disasters happen. Harriet's and Claire's relationship improves some, although they'll never again be close. Claire continues to manage Harriet's finances. Over time, Harriet's needs increase, and Susan ups her hours. She cooks Harriet's meals, helps her with toileting and bathing. Harriet faces an increasing risk of falling and hurting herself. Eventually, Susan, the aide, moves in with Harriet full-time. At night, she helps Harriet to the bathroom and watches over her when she is restless. Before long, Susan becomes exhausted. With her mother's funds, Claire hires another aide, this one from an agency, who spells Susan during the day. In the coming year, the cost of Harriet's care will exceed $90,000.

Claire continues to hope her mother will agree to nursing-home care. Claire begins regularly telling her mother that she's running out of money. "We *were* running out," Claire says, "but we weren't that close." Claire also regularly tells her mother, "I think you need more help than you get at home."

To secure a spot in a nursing home, Harriet needs a physical exam from a doctor. Claire arranges for the meeting. Claire and Harriet sit alone that day in the doctor's exam room, waiting for him to show up. A breakthrough happens: Harriet arrives at a "moment of clarity," Claire says. Harriet seems, momentarily, to return to her former, rational, reasonable self—"my old mom." Yes, Harriet says, she knows the current scenario isn't working. By now her memory and thinking have been seriously impaired by vascular dementia—the same sort of ongoing, small strokes that have damaged Mary's brain. The doctor's exam confirms this.

During a mini-mental-status test, Harriet is "all over the place," Claire says. Harriet cites the year as 1921. But in conversation with the physician, Harriet acknowledges, again, that she can't stay home any longer.

This comes, to Claire, as an enormous relief. A few days later, Claire moves Harriet to one of the nursing homes in which Harriet had received rehab; it's the same place in which Claire's father had spent his final months. Harriet moves in on a Friday. Weeks before, Claire had made plans to go away. She departs for the weekend.

Back in town a few days later, Claire visits the nursing home. She finds Harriet sitting by the window of her ground-floor room, in a geri chair. The staff have wheeled Harriet there because they know that Harriet likes to gaze at the view of the landscaped courtyard beyond. Claire walks up to Harriet and says hello. The sight of her mother startles her: the right side of Harriet's body is newly paralyzed, the right side of her face slack, immobile. Harriet has had a major stroke.

Claire feels suddenly panicky, an urgent need to *do* something. "I'll be right back!" she says to her mother. She runs into the hall, toward the nearby nurses' station.

Both of her parents, Claire says, "were very clear about end-of-life issues." They "didn't want their lives to be unnecessarily prolonged; they didn't want to live incapacitated." Nevertheless, Claire's father had ended up in the nursing home with dementia, confused and sad. He'd cried often. The time he spent in the facility was "like a prison sentence for him," Claire says. "My dad 'did' nineteen months." Claire sees the end of her mother's life in the same terms: "She's having to serve the time."

When Harriet was admitted, she had a do-not-resuscitate order in place, for any case in which her heart or breathing stopped. She and Claire's father had written advance directives, back when they were well. Harriet's document had "very clear wording," Claire says, "about not extending her life when there is no dignity or quality of life." Claire would find these words helpful as she made decisions on her mother's behalf. Claire had instructed the nursing home not to send her mother to the hospital for any reason. Should her mother have a stroke, in other words, nothing should be done. Still, deciding in theory that this is how you want a facility to respond, and finding your mother half-paralyzed after your weekend away—these are two very different emotional scenarios.

The day she discovers her mother's new, deteriorated state, Claire finds herself in the hall, "freaking out," distraught, crying. She assumes that her mother has just had this stroke, is even in the midst of it now. Otherwise, Claire feels, the staff would have called her over the weekend to let her know. She first encounters the nurse manager, who follows Claire back into Harriet's room. The nurse gazes at Harriet and says to Claire, "Oh, yes. She's been like this all weekend. We thought that was how she was."

For days afterward, Claire is upset with the facility and also feels guilty, as if the move to the nursing home, which Claire had pushed for, had caused her mother's stroke. But before long, Claire lets go, at least, of her anger at the staff. She is grateful for the facility and admires the care they're able to give. Still, she experiences the place as a terrible purgatory—mostly for her mother, but for herself, as well. She edits, in conversations with friends, part of the facility's name—"center for extended care"—to "center for *extending life*." The question, for Claire, is, why extend it? Harriet spends her days in a geri chair and in diapers. "She can't sit up," Claire says. "She doesn't have the trunk strength to hold herself up. Her feet are swollen; she can't walk; she can't feed herself. All she can do is talk. Her quality of life is nonexistent."

"Does she know you?" I ask.

"No. She's totally around the bend." Harriet lives, Claire says, in a wild, unknowable land of delusion. Harriet tells Claire stories about her love life, her marriages, her new baby. Fortunately, Harriet seems to enjoy rather than be disturbed by her hallucinations. "She's happy," Claire says. "She's had a very active dating life. She really loves this one guy she's been dating." Harriet sits in her geri chair by the nurses' station. She points to a woman in a nearby chair and announces that she has had "a relationship" with her. She tells Claire that a CIA agent once came into her room and had sex with Harriet's roommate. Harriet refers to her boyfriends, variously, as Renee, Riley, "my chubby boyfriend," and "the three redheads."

When Claire visits, she doesn't say much to her mother. Claire pulls a chair from the nurses' station, places it next to her mother's geri chair, sits, and asks, "What's new?"—and listens to her mother's fantastical news.

When Harriet lived next door, Claire says, "I missed her *a lot*." Claire wanted, as she'd said back in August to the support group, her "old mother back." Now, "I'm used to her being gone. There's this woman in the nursing home I have a duty to. But she is unrecognizable to me as my mother. She doesn't look like my mother anymore; she doesn't have any of my mother's characteristics. It's like she's already died."

Final grief is suspended, and in-the-meantime grief goes on. "I wish for my mother's death. And I dread it, too." Claire pauses, her dark eyes looking at me over a cup of hot chocolate. "I think if there is a God, He should release my mother from the prison of her body."

. . .

The line between illness and dying, in Alzheimer's and other chronic, fatal, progressive diseases, is not bright, says Dr. Diane Meier, a professor of geriatrics and internal medicine at Mount Sinai School of Medicine, a MacArthur "genius" grant winner, and a fierce advocate for palliative care—"comfort care" for people facing serious illness and/or death. The line is much clearer, Meier says, in cancer, for example. We know cancer's narrative. Generally speaking, doctors and families recognize when the end is near: once a patient becomes bedridden, death is likely within a few months. But with dementia and other chronic, degenerative diseases, the end is much less predictable. Bedridden incapacity can go on for years.

Dementia patients tend to die in one of two ways, Meier says: In the first, death comes relatively suddenly in the midst of long, slow decline. The final, lethal event may be an infection in the lungs or urinary tract; it may be a heart attack, stroke, or fall. "Things are going along as usual," she says, "and then some acute crisis intervenes and the person doesn't have enough reserve anymore to bounce back." Death is "unexpected" in the sense that if the person hadn't fallen, hadn't gotten a cold, if his or her heart rhythm hadn't been disturbed, he or she would still be alive. The end is sudden, in the context of a life that has slowly been fading out.

With this type of death, the cause may be listed on the death certificate as heart failure or pneumonia, but the real cause can be seen as the underlying, fatal condition—a body and a brain that have long been failing. (This helps explain an undercounting of Alzheimer's deaths in official records.) "It's really hard to think of [dementia] as a terminal illness," Meier says, "when somebody's been living with it for years. But it *is* a terminal illness. Nobody gets better from dementia." It is therefore "hard to get a societal narrative that makes sense for the progress of dementia towards death. Everybody knows what to expect with cancer. The cognitive train for that is established." But dementia, she believes, from working with patients and families, "is not thought about as something you die from. It's thought about as something you live with."

Ours is an age of extraordinary, lifesaving medical interventions, which have enabled people to live much longer than they did a century ago. Yet at some point in illness, interventions come not only at great cost—both financially and in misery—they also become futile. Studies show that opting only for comfort care at the end of life, as Claire did for her mother, can actually extend life and make death more peaceful. Interventions that would once have saved a stronger person's life—a feeding tube, a respirator, or surgery—can shorten a frail person's life by causing stress and pain.

How to know when lifesaving measures should stop? Meier works to help her medical colleagues, as well as patients and families, make this decision well. It means, in large part, she says, physicians' fostering discussion with patients and families. A doctor caring for a person with a fatal illness, she says, should seek to understand the patient's and/or family's wishes and values, the extent to which the family grasps the nature and progression of the disease, and—once this understanding is reached—what treatments a family wants. When a patient has advanced dementia, a physician should ask, "If Mrs. Jones were sitting in the room with us, if she were able to return to her prior self and could be part of this conversation, what do you think she would be telling us right now?"

Meier says she typically hears one of three answers to this question. "She would never want to live like this" is the most common. The second is "I have no idea what she would want. We never talked about it." The third, "She made me promise to do everything possible to keep her alive as long as possible," is most common among the religious.

When a doctor does not encourage discussion, Meier says, caregivers can seek it themselves. They can ask the doctor, How will this disease progress? What are the options? Given my mother's wishes, what would you recommend?

For a year following Harriet's stroke, Claire visits her mother every few weeks. She can't bear to look in more often. Each time she does visit, she stops at the nurses' station and asks for a report on her mother's health. Staff call Harriet "stable." Claire hears the word so often that Harriet's condition comes to seem almost eternal. Small changes do happen. One day as Harriet sits slumped in her geri chair, telling stories, Claire spots decay in her mother's teeth. It distresses Claire. Later she asks the nursing home what can be done. A dentist does visit the home occasionally and tend to the residents' mouths, but Claire learns that getting her mother this care will be complicated.

It happens that Claire has spotted the tooth problem only days before Harriet dies. Hearing the story later, after Harriet's death, I ask Claire how she had felt about her mother's teeth: Was she worried that her mother was in pain? That she couldn't eat? Claire says she can't pinpoint her attitude. Her mother was being fed puréed food, so eating wasn't the issue. Harriet didn't seem to be in pain. Claire was simply acting as she felt she should. "I wasn't thinking, 'Oh, we might as well not deal with her teeth because she's going to die soon.' It was just like, 'That's what you do for people; you take care of their teeth.'"

In this age of slow loss, a typical twenty-first-century narrative of elder caregiving has emerged. For a period, possibly a long one, a daughter may take care of her mother's finances. A wife may drive because her husband no longer can. A son may do his father's grocery shopping. A charge's abilities decrease, and a caregiver's duties increase commensurately. Eventually, we imagine, near-complete impairment sets in, a person becomes bedridden, perhaps moves to a nursing home for round-the-clock care, or invites a hospice program into the home. The caregiver's own response adapts as needed. In a last, intense period, the caregiver oversees professional care and/or provides for a loved one's needs. Then comes a final slide to death.

But the details are never entirely predictable. Decline surprises; it happens in fits and spurts—health stabilizes, takes another dive, plateaus again. Relationships change: caregivers themselves become ill or divorce their spouses or die. Uncertainty makes planning difficult. Perhaps a patient's insurance entitles her to only a month of hospice care. How to know when the patient is precisely that far from death? It is almost impossible *to* know. Sometimes, as Meier describes in the first type of death with dementia, the end comes suddenly after years of slow decline.

Sometimes it seems as if the end will never arrive. This sort of endless end constitutes the second type of death caused by dementia and other chronic, progressive brain diseases—an "excruciatingly slow process of gradual decline," Meier says. The brain slowly and inexorably continues to lose function. All the body's processes shut down, in nearly the reverse order in which a person made gains at the beginning of life: the brain can no longer instruct the body to walk, sit up, eat, swallow, and, finally, breathe. "You don't do any of those things consciously," Meier says. "They just happen because your brain is functioning." When the brain doesn't work, nothing else will.

This kind of death, Meier says, while "in some ways easier to prepare for, at least in theory, is also very difficult because it's so prolonged. It's not like the family can come in and do the vigil, and we can say, 'Your mom is likely to be dead in a week or two.' The family can come in and do the vigil, and the vigil can go on for months."

Claire's mother will die the first way—relatively suddenly. One Saturday morning, Claire finds several messages on her cell phone. Staff have called to say that Harriet's condition has quickly deteriorated. They believe Harriet has had another major stroke; she is running a low fever; she likely has pneumonia. They seem to know that this is the beginning of the end for Harriet. Still, it takes Claire a long time for the phone messages to "sink in." She drives her daughter to a birthday party, makes arrangements for her ride home, runs a few errands. Finally, in the afternoon, Claire heads to the nursing home. She finds her mother in bed, propped up so that her breathing will be easier. Claire can see that her mother *has* had another stroke: for the first time, Harriet is unable to take food or speak. Harriet tries occasionally to say things, but no words form. What strikes Claire more than anything, however, is that her mother seems more aware, even content, than before: she smiles each time someone enters her room.

Claire begins the first of two vigils by her mother's bedside. "I don't know how [the nursing-home staff] know" that a resident is approaching death, Claire says. She assumes they've learned signs—breathing changes, unresponsiveness, some predictable series of subtle events. In the late afternoon, with Harriet going in and out of semiconsciousness, Claire leaves the facility; she drives her children to a theater performance she'd long ago bought tickets for. Claire will remember nothing of the show. She is "completely on another planet," thinking of her mother, knowing she will soon die. Claire takes her children home; everyone goes to bed. Claire makes sure she has a phone at her bedside. It rings at four in the morning: it's getting close to time, a nurse says. Claire pads down the hall and wakes her son, now fifteen. "I'm going to the nursing home," she says. "Grandma is dying."

She pulls up to the facility in the dark. In her mother's room, Claire draws a chair up to Harriet's bed. A nurse offers tea and fruit. Claire doesn't feel hungry. Soon a neighbor, a friend of both Claire's and her mother's, arrives and sits by Claire. Claire watches her mother in bed. Harriet's face is slack, unmoving, her mouth slightly open—Claire is not sure whether to consider it "expressionless" or fixed in a painful grimace. She wonders about the experience of dying. The nurses have begun giving Harriet liquid morphine, squirted with a needle-less syringe between her lips. Claire is glad for the narcotic, often given to the dying to relieve pain and—an unspoken goal—perhaps help death come more easily. She listens to her mother's breathing, hard and fast. Harriet is pulling in air, apparently desperately, but Claire can't know for sure. She remembers that her father breathed this way, too, toward his end. Back then, she yearned to know if her father understood that Claire was there with him. But here with her mother, Claire doesn't feel as strong an urge to know. She is simply attending her mother's death—for her own sake, but also in case she does, by her presence, provide her mother with solace.

Listening to her mother breathe, it strikes Claire that Harriet is laboring, that this dying is hard work. Perhaps her mother is already "gone," and this breathing is simply the body's—the brain stem's—refusal to give in. On the other hand, who knows, her mother may be aware she is dying, in which case, Claire believes, Harriet is "fighting to let go"—a strange paradox.

Midmorning, and quite suddenly, Harriet's breathing changes; it slows and quiets. Claire remembers that this shift had happened in her father, too, just before he'd died. She turns to her neighbor and says, "Now she's actively dying." Claire takes her mother's hand. It feels, at once, clammy and warm—and surprisingly bony.

There is so little muscle left; for a long time Harriet has done nothing with her hands.

"It's okay to go," Claire murmurs to her mother. Soon she says it again.

I ask Meier how she defines a "good death."

"Families," Meier says, "define it for you." She hears, generally, one of two reactions from families to their loved ones' deaths. In the regrettable scenarios, family members say, "It was terrible. She was in a tremendous amount of pain." These relatives have been through great stress. They avoid eye contact with Meier; they show signs of guilt and embarrassment. "They feel like they've failed their loved ones," she says. "It's very hard to recover from a death when families feel like they weren't able to secure the right care"—that they didn't do right by their charges. Caregivers who have witnessed difficult deaths tend to grieve longer and experience greater rates of post-traumatic stress, Meier says.

Meier strives for the better scenarios, the ones in which family members say a death was "very peaceful," that their loved one experienced no pain, and that "we were all there." These survivors "go on to heal and recover," Meier says. In these cases, she says, "I know I did a good job."

Survivors face a much higher risk of trauma after their loved ones have died in hospitals, particularly intensive care units. They have a lower risk of trauma if their charges died at home with hospice care, or in nursing homes. Meier has spent much of her career working to convince her fellow physicians that they must help families secure palliative care, help them decide when to stop interventions, and help people die without pain. Failing at this not only "waste[s] shared precious resources, but actually does great harm" to survivors, for years afterward. "We have," she says, "a responsibility for that."

. . .

Claire says that what lingers painfully in her mind is not the short period during which her mother precipitously declined and died. Claire feels no guilt about that; she knew what her mother wanted, and she carried those wishes through. It is the longer descent, including the year in which her mother "did time" in the nursing home—alive, but not herself—that troubles Claire. This period, the death before death, seems like a larger, abstract injustice that doesn't have an answer. Short of assisting with suicide, no doctor could prevent it.

Part of her pain, Claire says, is that with long, slow loss, it's impossible to know when to say good-bye. She thinks back to that moment in the physician's office, when she was alone with her mother, the moment in which Harriet was lucid. "That was the last time I spent with my mother as I knew her. To me, that [moment] was good-bye. After that, I never saw my old mom, the one who raised me, and who I loved." Her mother's final death, then, came both hard and as a relief. Twenty minutes after her breathing had changed that morning, after Claire had recognized the signs, Harriet exhaled for the last time. Claire was still holding her hand.

Leisel

Inga invites me to go with her one evening to the college's arts center to hear a social-work professor give a lecture about grief. We sit at the front of a small, dimly lit theater. The professor suggests that our usual thinking about loss is inadequate. The death of a loved one, she says, is more than a terrible event that we eventually get over. The professor's sister had died a few years before, of cancer.

From this experience, the professor became convinced that grief can be transformative—that mourners create important meaning out of loss. They find ways to carry forward the values and passions of the deceased—through memorials, even social action. They create ways to maintain, within their psyches, relationships with those who are gone. Psychotherapists increasingly challenge the idea that successful mourning requires "getting over it" within a defined time frame. Rather, the challenge is to live well *within* grief, to integrate the loss into one's psyche and life's work. Grief, the professor says, can transform the mourner in unexpected and positive ways.

After the lecture, walking out, Inga says, "Well, *that* was an affirmation of experience!" During the talk, she had been thinking, "*I* could have written this."

"You're an expert," I say.

"Yes."

Inga's daughter, Leisel, was fifteen when Louise and Inga first got together. Over the following years, the two women increasingly parented Leisel together. Leisel grew into an independent and accomplished person. She edited her high school's literary magazine, had many friends, graduated sixth in her high school class. She received a scholarship to George Washington University, where she edited the college's literary review and founded a tutoring program for inner-city children.

She once told Inga and Louise that their biggest fault as parents was that they didn't provide enough constraints to rebel against. She felt almost hampered by her freedom. This isn't to say Inga and Louise were permissive mothers. They had strong ideas about independence and initiative. They required Leisel to go to a college at least 150 miles away, and that she work while there. In a letter to Leisel during her first year of college, Inga writes, *I hope you'll . . . recognize that this planned schedule for no-nonsense living is the proper way to make the most of your many and diverse skills and talents. I am very much in favor of your trying out for the next play. Being in theater develops your poise, self-confidence and appreciation for yourself and others.*

Later in the same letter, Inga writes, *The task of developing greater consideration and respect is another to tackle promptly. . . . I agree that you've been spoiled in a few ways. I still won't admit that you're [truly] spoiled because I can point with pride to such things as your being willing, even excited, about wearing a secondhand coat. Anyway, Louise loves spending money on you, but you'll have to say or do some things to make sure you indicate you don't take it for granted. . . .*

Do excellently! Take the best care of your body and mind that is possible. You'll need both of them for a long, wonderful future.

Your ToughLove Mother, Inga writes. She signs the letter with the Norwegian word for mother, Leisel's pet name for her—*Mor.*

After college, Leisel moved to Richmond, Virginia. She worked as a graphic designer and volunteered in community theater. In the spring of 1989, she developed a cold that wouldn't go away. A doctor first advised patience, treating it as a stubborn virus. Leisel attended a cast party on a Friday night, feeling ill. She felt no better by Monday and returned to the doctor. The physician ordered blood tests. The results were alarming. The doctor told Leisel to head straight to the Medical College of Virginia for more tests. Leisel left Inga a message at the school where Inga taught, and Inga called back.

"I have an elevated white blood cell count," Leisel said. "Am I going to be hospitalized?"

"Probably," Inga said.

An oncologist called Inga the next day during Inga's lunch break: "I've just diagnosed your daughter with acute myeloid leukemia." He wanted to begin treatment that day.

Inga and Louise decided that Leisel should stay in Virginia for her medical care. Inga took a leave from her job. "This was before the Family Leave Act," she says, but she and Louise were lucky. They could afford Inga's taking time off. Inga moved to Richmond. For the next six months, she lived in an executive apartment and spent most of her waking hours with Leisel at the hospital. Louise flew south every weekend and joined them. "Out" lesbian couples were hardly common in Virginia during that time. A nurse who at first acted coldly toward the couple eventually said, "If you three aren't a family, I don't know who is."

Leisel had an aggressive form of leukemia. But "everyone kept telling her that she would survive it," Louise says. Leisel was young and had been in excellent health. She endured her first chemotherapy treatment, and a second. The cancer did not respond. An oncologist said to Inga, "You understand we do not cure AML here?"

Inga said, "Yes, we're hoping for a remission." The doctor nodded. Still, Inga says, everyone was operating on the belief that "miracles happen."

Inga learned as much as she could about Leisel's disease. "I latched on to student nurses." One of them helped Inga get access to the medical library. During the day, "when Leisel was sleeping, I would rush over to the library and sit and read—everything I could in all the medical journals—about leukemia." The news she found there, Inga says, was "miserable." AML had a slim long-term survival rate. "I'd put on my face and go back" to Leisel's room.

Early on, Inga resolved to maintain her composure and, if not optimism, at least as positive an attitude as she could muster. Inga taped a sign to the wall of Leisel's room: YOU CAN'T AFFORD THE

LUXURY OF A NEGATIVE THOUGHT. Leisel sometimes pointed to it if she sensed the atmosphere in the room was turning maudlin. "We would, in effect, buck up and cope," Inga says. She remembers several days during which she shared "a lot of tears" with Leisel—"when we knew that unfinished business had to be discussed and aired, before there was no more opportunity to do that." But Inga says that most days, she allowed herself only ten minutes to cry, in the morning before she left the apartment. "Then I put on my game face and drove to the hospital." At night, she spent a couple of hours on the phone, updating family and friends (this was before mass e-mails and personal websites). She read books she'd checked out of the public library, "anything and everything I could find on leukemia; on grieving as a parent; death and dying of any variety. I even checked out children's books. I remember one called *Freddie the Leaf.* I would read myself to sleep."

Inga sought support from colleagues, friends, family. "I wrote to everybody and told them exactly what was going on and what I needed. Whatever they came up with, it helped to sustain me." Although often there was no obvious way that the support—gifts, cards, phone calls—eased Inga's burdens, the gestures gave her mental strength.

"In the hospital room, we maximized the good days. We searched for ways to laugh. We rented comedy tapes. We borrowed the newspaper comic pages. I wrote to the jokester in our school: 'Tommy,' I said, 'please, I need jokes—good ones, bad ones—just send jokes.' He did. I sat there reading them, and Leisel laughed—so much that the head nurse came in and said, 'You people are having entirely too much fun in here; it's upsetting everybody.'

"But we had to," Inga says. "It was so *grim.* So unbelievably grim."

· · ·

Leisel received two more rounds of chemotherapy. The cancer was unaffected. By midsummer, she had grown too frail, her physicians felt, to survive a fifth. Inga arranged for a train trip—flying carried too great an infection risk—north to Washington, DC. Leisel said good-bye to old friends.

During her treatments, Leisel contracted hepatitis C from a blood transfusion. (The virus was then called "non-A, non-B hepatitis." There was no way to test for it in the blood supply.) The virus would end her life. There was no cure. When the news came back that Leisel had the disease, her doctors, Inga says, "just couldn't face the fact that they didn't have an answer to it." (In a few years, more effective treatments would be found.) With the cancer not responding to treatments, and hepatitis on top of it, Inga realized that the time had come to make hard decisions.

"While she was still competent, very early in the month of September, before she had lost her ability to write, I talked to one of the nurses I was closest to." Inga told the nurse that she wanted to help Leisel put her end-of-life wishes in writing. "I want Leisel to be the one who discusses, understands, and signs it," Inga said.

The nurse nodded. "I can help you with that."

"So she got the paperwork, and she and I sat down with Leisel." Inga explained to her daughter that hepatitis C was incurable. She told Leisel that her doctors would be able only to treat infections, as they had been doing all along. "Do you understand?"

"Yeah. All I'd like to know is how long will it take." Leisel meant, how long before I die?

Inga told Leisel, "We'll find that out. You deserve answers." Inga says that she described to Leisel the advance directive they had prepared. The doctors will "want to keep pumping things into you, because they're trained that way. But this paper tells them, 'If I can't recover, stop it. But keep me from having pain, even if it means that I go into a semiconscious state.'"

Leisel listened, and signed the form.

Inga says, "It was as if from that day on, she allowed herself to begin to die." Along the way, Leisel finally got angry. She was so weak that she could express her anger only by throwing paper airplanes across the room. Soon she stopped eating. But "about two weeks before she died," Inga says, Leisel asked for pizza. Inga drove around town, looking for a restaurant that made it. "Pizza was not common in Richmond" at the time. She drove "into this horrible section of town," the wrong way down a one-way street, and found a place with "pizza that looked to me like the sorriest thing in the world." She drove a pizza back to the hospital. Leisel chewed a few bites and, unable to swallow by this time, spit them out again. "That was the last food she ate. Or rather, tasted. Poor child."

Doctors provided Leisel with a self-administered morphine pump. The nurses, Inga says, paid close attention to how much morphine Leisel was using. They provided records of the use to doctors and let the physicians know if they believed Leisel wasn't getting enough medication—if they suspected that Leisel was in pain. The nurses told Inga to watch for signs of suffering. If Leisel "can't remember to push the button for the morphine, you do it," they told Inga. "She asked not to be in pain. This is what we can do."

One Saturday in mid-October, Inga says, the physicians decided to put a central line into a vein in Leisel's neck. All of the veins in her hands and feet and arms were, Inga says, "completely blown." Louise, who had flown down from Long Island, sent Inga out of Leisel's room. "Go to a museum or take a walk," Louise said. She wanted to spare Inga the pain of witnessing another procedure. Inga left. Louise waited down the hall. She remembers hearing screams from Leisel's room.

A resident "did get the central line in," Inga says. "But it clogged up right away," so the clinician took it out again. The team finally halted all measures. "They said, 'Okay. We're going to stop. We're going to stop.'"

That night, not knowing how long Leisel would live, Inga and

Louise went home to sleep a little. The next morning, Louise felt antsy. "We *have* to get to the hospital," Inga remembers Louise saying. "No stopping for coffee or breakfast." They arrived on Leisel's unit a little before eight. Louise went straight from the elevator to Leisel's room. Inga stopped at the nurses' station, as usual, to ask a nurse how Leisel had fared overnight. She learned that Leisel had been unconscious, breathing slowly.

Louise called Inga from the doorway to Leisel's room: "Inga, get in here. Now."

A moment later, Inga walked into her daughter's room. Gaunt, eyes closed, wearing one of the many scarves that had been made for her, Leisel lay in a "state-of-the-art" hospital bed, as Inga calls it, that monitored heart rate and respiration without wires. Louise had lain down on the far side of Leisel's bed, by the windows. Inga walked across the room, retracted the bed rail, and lay next to Leisel on the bed's near side. She remembers hearing only the sound of her daughter breathing. She placed her hand on Leisel's chest. "It's okay," Inga whispered. "You can go safely. I love you. Your grandpas will be there. It will be okay." Inga says, "We talked her through good-bye."

At eight fifteen, Leisel took her last breath.

While in the hospital, Leisel had written a poem for Inga, secretly giving it to Louise, asking her to present it to Inga on Mother's Day the following year. The poem included the lines: *I go to the unknown in the beyond. I will always and forever be at your side.*

For years afterward, each morning upon waking, Inga pictured Leisel beside her. "I have you *here*," she thought to herself. Describing this, Inga gestures beside her. She doesn't imagine Leisel *within* her, she says. Her daughter remains separate, yet present. Leisel, in this way, keeps Inga company.

After Leisel's death, Inga struggled not to let the loss destroy her. She is a resourceful, practical person and turned these qualities to learning how to endure grief. She consulted a therapist, joined support groups. She founded an award in Leisel's honor at Leisel's old high school. Every year for two decades, until recently, Inga has traveled to the school and introduced the grant. She has witnessed its presentation to the year's honoree, a student chosen for his or her promise in writing and academic achievement.

One of the support groups Inga joined after Leisel's death was for parents who had lost children. She listened to their stories and felt grateful. At least she'd had time with Leisel between Leisel's diagnosis and death. "I learned that if your child had to die, it certainly was a lot better to go through six months of intense *life* with her, while you learned how to say good-bye, than it was to cope with a suicide, an automobile accident," or other sudden death.

Inga also followed a therapist's advice: "Do for and with others that which I hoped for in life with Leisel." She and Leisel had planned to drive cross-country together one day. Instead, Inga took her mother to Norway for two weeks. She bought a condominium for her mother. Leisel had always enthusiastically celebrated holidays, so Inga organized for her mother "a seventy-fifth birthday bash" and an "eightieth birthday bash."

Inga has relied, throughout her losses, on a mix of practicality and faith—not religion so much as a trust in some larger, unifying force, a basic goodness. She has sought out the resources she needs, as she puts it, "to find strength and carry on." Every year on the anniversary of Leisel's death, Inga lights a candle and remembers. She sends a memorial e-mail to friends and family. This fall of 2010, the twenty-first anniversary of Leisel's passing, Inga's e-mail includes the line *In my dreams, I search for the unfinished art of your life*. She signs the message *Mor*.

"It was a profound experience, a life-changing experience," Inga says. "To lose one's only child is its own thing." I ask Inga about her experience of fear in caregiving. She fixes me with her deep blue eyes. "I have no fear. It disappeared when my daughter died."

From the day of Leisel's death, Louise says, "We had a totally different way of looking at our lives." Before long, Louise had taken an early retirement. She and Inga decided they would do what they wanted; they would "do life." They took trips nearly every month for a year.

Louise's string of health problems began too soon after that. But the women's shared philosophy remained "Grab life; don't let it go." Louise says, "Inconsequential things *do* become inconsequential."

In the year since her recovery from MRSA, and in response to her other illnesses, Louise says, her attitude has shifted some. "Doing life" has evolved into "just being." She often sits in a rocker out on their deck. Inga asks her, "What are you doing?"

Louise replies, "I'm *being*."

But Inga finds herself still doing. After intensive caregiving, coping, and persevering, it is challenging for Inga to "just be." Part of this, Inga says, is that she still sees herself as "living in the world for both my daughter and myself."

There is twice as much to see and do.

Redemption

In mid-September 2010, the first cool and bright day of the fall arrives, winter-jacket cold. For a couple of weeks, feeble rain has fallen occasionally, but lawns still crackle underfoot; leaves are still shrunken and brittle.

On weekends, Penny has driven along roads in her area, scanned woods, pulled over at promising spots, and collected seeds for an international seed exchange in which the college participates. On the path of a Connecticut canal, she stretches over her head into a sassafras tree, but can't reach the dark specks she has spied among the leaves. She sees a man and woman walking toward her with three dogs. The man is very tall, perhaps seven feet. Ordinarily, on these outings, Penny says, she keeps to herself. But the man's height, she realizes, could come in handy. She calls hello, and the couple stop. They ask what she's doing. Penny tells them and pulls a few leaves off the sassafras tree. "They're unusual," she says. See the three types?

She offers tastes. "Refreshing, huh?" she asks of the root-beer-like flavor. They agree.

Penny says to the man, "You know, I bet you could reach that branch up there without jumping." As it turns out, he does have to jump a little, but he grabs the branch and pulls it down. Penny plucks seeds and thanks him.

Late in September, a deluge comes—walls of water in sudden, furious downpours. Basements flood around town, and water trickles into a room near Penny's office. The rain continues off and on into October. Streams and rivers fill, and the grass turns green for a last show of color before the freeze. Trees brighten. Reds and oranges flare along wooded roadways.

One September day, Penny says to the group, "I got really angry with my mom yesterday." Penny had stopped at an Italian pastry shop on her way home from work. "My mom is prediabetic so she doesn't get sugar very often," Penny reminds everyone. As a rare treat, Penny says, she bought two cannoli.

She walked into the house with the pastries in a bag and said to Mary, "I brought dessert!"

They ate dinner, and Penny told her mother that later they

would indulge. Penny left the bag in the kitchen and drove to an AA meeting.

When she returned, the treats had gone missing. She scanned the counters, opened cabinets. Gazing from the kitchen into the living room, she spied the paper bag, lying crumpled "as if a dog or something had gotten into it," on the thigh-high chest behind the couch, where Mary was sitting. Penny walked over, picked up the bag, and said, "Oh, Mom, *here* it is!"

Penny heard a small, meek voice coming from the couch: *"I ate both of them."*

The group laughs, and Penny does, too. But at the time, she says, "I was so angry I couldn't be in the same room with her." She went to the back of the house and wrote wrathful e-mails to her sister and a friend. "When I get that mad, I want to get revenge. I think about the ways I could punish her, like, *No dessert. Ever again.*" Penny felt frustrated, betrayed.

She thinks about a story she heard at an AA meeting: "This guy took care of puppies when he was little. He loved puppies. He had a litter of them to take care of, and every morning he had to clean up the by-product of the puppies. It didn't bother him because, he said, 'That's the nature of puppies.'"

"I know she's not a puppy," Penny says, but she hears in the story a message about accepting what and whom you cannot change, about understanding the reasons for others' behavior.

Still, she wants to say to Mary, *"No cannoli in my house. Ever again!"*

"Like the Soup Nazi," Ben says, recalling the television show *Seinfeld.*

"That's exactly how I felt." Penny told her mother that "part of her" wanted to say, "We should not have dessert in the house ever again."

"And my mom said"—Penny again imitates the small, meek voice—"'What does the *other* part say?'"

"Aaaaw," a newcomer says sympathetically from down the table.

William, who has for years been witnessing impulsive behavior at the nursing home, says, "Most of the patients start with their dessert anyway. There are a couple of them who take sugar packets and open them up and . . ." He mimes pouring sugar into his mouth.

Penny nods and sighs. That night, she says, she awoke, startled, from a dream. Her father, gone for more than five years, had appeared in the dream. He was not well, but alive. "Back from the dead," Penny says. "My mother was so happy to see him. But I was like, 'Oh my God. He's going to *die* again! What are we going to do with the body?'"

The next morning, Penny called Sophie, told her about the dream, and cried. Penny was feeling, again, the fear of losing their mother. The evening before, Penny had complained to Sophie about the cannoli. That morning Sophie said, referring to the dream and to Penny's anger the night before, "Maybe it was Dad coming back to say, 'Hey, take it easy, Penny. She's going to be with me before you know it.'"

Penny tells the group that she recently watched a documentary film made in the 1990s by a woman who was struggling to care for her addled mother. The film was called *Complaints of a Dutiful Daughter.*

Ben asks, "So are you a dutiful daughter?"

"Um. I'm doing way better than that woman in the film. But it's at my own expense. I don't think they had caregiver support groups back then." As for *complaints,* there is always something to grumble about. "If it's out there, I'm going to find it."

"You're a dog with a bone," Ben says, using one of Penny's favorite expressions.

Penny chuckles. "Yeah! And I'm going to let people know." For example, yesterday she arrived home and found a voice message from a company that once supplied the oxygen concentrator for Mary's CPAP mask. The message said the company needed to come and pick up the device. *"Guess what,"* Penny says to the group, "they picked it up back in *April*." This sort of sudden and confusing event agitates her, gets her mind spinning. She was thinking, Medicare fraud, and, Strange men coming into my house without my knowing.

She asked her mother, "Did they come into the house?"

Mary, of course, couldn't remember.

"So I was getting all paranoid," Penny says to the group. "Who are these people? What are they going to do to my mother?"

Penny smiles, remembering what happened next. She called the company's toll-free number. "I got Sean in *Bombay*."

Everyone laughs at this familiar, global-economy scenario.

Sean was unable to give Penny useful information. Penny said, "You know what, Sean? I think maybe I should talk to somebody more *local*." Sean obliged, and Penny found herself speaking with a woman in Tennessee. The woman searched her database and found a few outdated notes about Mary's account, but no answers regarding the oxygen concentrator. "So I was thinking," Penny says, "I have to go *more* local. I'm going to call the number I should have called in the first place." She punched digits and reached someone in her own area code.

She learned that the company had neglected to end the service contract on the oxygen concentrator. There had been an error of record keeping.

"That's all I wanted to hear!" Penny says to the group. "That somebody made a mistake. At first they wouldn't admit it. But I said, 'So somebody made a mistake.'" The woman on the phone said, "'Yep, that's what happened.' I said, 'Okay! I'm satisfied!'"

"Penny, you're stomping on those ANTs," Ben says.

Penny considers. "Yeah. Well, is that a good thing?"

"Yeah. Your paranoia went away." Ben points out that Penny acted on her fear: she investigated the situation and got resolution.

"Yeah," Penny says. "But wouldn't it be nice if the fear didn't just go *ping* right from the start?"

In September, Penny celebrates her fiftieth birthday. On her calendar, in the square designating her birth date, Penny writes, *25 x 2!*

Ben brings to the group a cake decorated with Penny's name. Everyone passes around pieces of cake, and Penny reads the card that people have signed. When it is her turn to share, she looks around and says, "Thank you so much. I really appreciate what you all said." She looks down the table at Daniel. "Thanks, Daniel." He nods and tips his cap.

She tells everyone that she is still struggling with how long it will be before she moves her mother to assisted living. "I had another meltdown yesterday at work." A coworker, whose mother lives in an assisted-living facility, stood in front of Penny, held her hands, looked Penny in the eye, and said, "Penny, you're going to have to come to terms." The woman meant that Penny is going to have to face, head-on, when she'll move Mary elsewhere.

"I said to her, 'I know. I've got the paperwork. I just can't sit down and fill out the form. I just don't want to do it.'"

Into the fall, Liz endures a six-week recovery from her illness. Doctors say she shouldn't drive. She doesn't mind skipping her visits to Joe at the veterans home, but she misses babysitting her grandson, Liam. She frets about how she will get to doctors' and psychotherapy appointments, and the caregivers' meetings. She consults

Sarah from the group. Sarah and Liz are becoming friends. Sarah has been calling Liz regularly and checking in. Sarah suggests getting rides from the senior center's van. "I feel like I'm ninety," Liz says to me. "Calling a van from the *senior* center for a ride!" She sighs. "I tell you, Nell. Make the best of each day, while you're young."

I give her a ride to the hospital on a Thursday for a chest X-ray. We'll go to the support-group meeting afterward. Liz sits in the waiting room near the hospital's lobby. We chat.

She says she has heard that caregivers often die before their charges do because of stress. Listening to Liz, I think of what Suzanne Mintz, executive director of the National Family Caregivers Association, said to me in an interview: "I think watching someone you love deteriorate is really more stress than anything in the world." Perhaps just as much, or even more so, when it is someone you no longer love, but feel obligated to.

Stress is almost always at least an implicit topic in the support group. At one meeting in October, members discuss it in a particularly direct way. First Penny talks about her frustration with Meals-On-Wheels. Many of the meals contain too much sodium for Mary. A blood test recently showed that Mary's heart was working too hard, perhaps because of elevated sodium in her blood.

Miriam—the woman whose husband, James, died a year ago of Parkinson's, and who drops into the meetings about once a month—interjects, looking around the table through her cat-eye glasses, "It's such a big issue for caregivers. Some of the things that are designed to help us are more trouble than doing it ourselves. I'm throwing this out as an issue for all of us: In what ways can we make use of services without injuring ourselves further?" Having James in a nursing home at the end of his life "was an *additional* stress on me." When he was home, she felt she had control— over his medications, their timing, the food James ate, and so on. "Once he was up there, if they made a mistake, I went ballistic." She pauses. "But what was the point? I was killing myself." Looking back after his death, she realized she had expected she could keep him alive.

Not long after James died, Miriam was besieged with her own health problems. She had several strokes and later a pulmonary embolism. More recently, she has been diagnosed with polycythemia, a blood disorder. She tells the group that her doctor has told her that the blood disorder is due to an acquired mutation in a gene—and that stress may have caused the mutation.

"Miriam," Penny says, "do you want to hear something? This means we have control issues. This is what it means."

"But, thank God we *have* control!"

"Well, yes and no," Penny says. "Because, you know, you were stressing yourself out."

Penny saw her own doctor the day before. Penny talked with her physician about the strain of overseeing what her mother eats. The doctor encouraged Penny to relax a little: "Penny, you're putting yourself in your mother's place. You're not the prediabetic. She is. She's *eighty-seven*. This is not about *life expectancy*. It's about keeping her comfortable and happy." Penny says she found this advice helpful. The comment changed her perspective; she felt a little more calm. "It doesn't seem like it today. I'm ready to cry. But it made me think, 'Okay, just chill out.' Because there are only so many things you can control." Penny narrows her eyes. "I just don't always have the *wisdom to know the difference*."

Miriam concedes, "We're not going to stand between our loved person and the inevitable. We're not going to stand between that person and the development of their disease or their final demise. And yet, there are so many things that, by being in control, we *do* make better for them." She pauses. "But it's at our expense."

Penny nods. "Do no harm," she says in an apparent attempt to sum things up.

In informal caregiving, finding a way to entirely avoid harm, to both caregiver and recipient, can feel nearly, or entirely, impossible. It is one thing to hold the intention, another to execute the ideal. Perhaps "Do the most good and least harm possible, given imperfect circumstances" is a more achievable aim. Inga remembers her mother saying, toward the end of her life, "I've gotten this far. I'm going to eat what I want, get out of the house when I can, and sleep when I can. So be it." She was focusing on quality of life rather than length. Later, in the parking lot of the hospital, Penny talks again about not treating her mother's life span as the ultimate measure of caregiving success. Penny says that when her uncle Gerald was dying in a nursing home, the staff wouldn't allow him to eat honey, which he loved. "Even on the day he *died*!" Penny pauses, considering her mother's situation. "So maybe we should start eating bacon again." On second thought, maybe *she,* Penny, shouldn't eat bacon. Her mom, though, might be allowed the enjoyment of it. The point is, Penny's outlook on her mother's health and longevity could shift a little. Penny smiles. Her friend Daphne would say, "Your mom's on another plane of existence, Penny. Let her be."

At another meeting in the fall, Penny tells the group that she has learned a technique for helping her mother with her confusion. Mary asks Penny over and over, as Penny is getting ready to leave the house, "Where're you going again?"

Penny says to the group, "So before I go, I write a little note." It tells Mary where Penny is heading and when she'll be back. Penny tapes it to Mary's walker. "If I put that on her cart before I leave, and she asks me again, I say, 'I think I put that on your cart.'"

Mary says, "Oh, that's right. It's there."

Ben says, "It comforts her."

"Yeah."

Penny thinks again of her uncle Gerald, who was blind and demented in the last years of his life. He relied, she says, on a device that regularly announced the day and time. But before he was given this tool, Penny says, "He would always ask me." All the time.

A new member nods. Her mother does the same thing.

Penny smiles. She used to say to her uncle, "It's two minutes since the *last* time you asked!" But this was, she knows now, "a smart-aleck thing to say," and not particularly kind. She pauses, reflecting. "I think I'm better now."

Ben nods. Earlier in the meeting, he had handed out a sheet that showed the group's growth in size, with the dates on which each member had first attended. "I think you're much better," he says, glancing at the sheet, "than you were on February twelfth, 2009."

Penny laughs. She wraps up her stories about the stresses of caregiving. Her mom is basically fine. "She's happy. A happy little Buddha."

"It's funny," Ben muses, chin in hand. "There's all this chaos. Your mom, she's like this solid nucleus of calm—with an atomic bomb going off around her."

"Yeah." Penny nods. It's true.

❧ "Something Snapped"

For months, Leanne has been "very volatile in her moods," Daniel says. She has said to Daniel, "I wish I were dead. All the pills would stop. All the problems would go away. You wouldn't have to take care of me." This fall he reports on continued swings in her mood and their marriage. He tells the group that he and Leanne had recently had a brief and honest exchange. "I know I'm difficult," Leanne said. "But so are you."

"I know I am," Daniel had replied. "But you're much *more* difficult."

Daniel chuckles and shakes his head, telling the story. Perhaps his finding humor in the situation gives the group permission to do the same. They laugh. "She didn't deny it," Daniel says, smiling, and the group laughs more.

"Beautiful," Ben says.

"That's what you call compatibility!" Inga says.

Later, Daniel says, he and Leanne found themselves giggling together at the kitchen table. Leanne said to Daniel, "We're not getting along, but we tell each other jokes that we like"—a sort of compatibility, too.

In mid-October, I miss a support-group meeting. On the phone with Penny later, I learn that Daniel had delivered difficult news: a few days before, Leanne had attempted suicide by taking an overdose of her medications. She had been admitted to Ben's ward.

Two weeks later, Daniel returns to the group. Ben is unable to attend. Only the married couples—Karen and Don, and a new pair, Linda and David—and Rufus, William, and Daniel show up. Daniel reports that Leanne is back home. He says he believes that one conflict in his marriage may, in part, have spurred her suicide attempt: she felt hurt by a long-distance, platonic friendship of Daniel's. He and a fellow academic had been talking on the phone and exchanging e-mails, mostly about scholarly and intellectual topics. Daniel had found the rapport with her enlivening. But, he tells everyone, he has ended the friendship, at Leanne's request.

A lively discussion ensues. Karen and Linda rue Daniel's decision; they believe that Daniel should pursue any friendship that nurtures him, as long as it doesn't violate his marriage vows. "We want you to be *happy*," Linda says. But the men—Rufus, William, and Don (Linda's husband, who has Alzheimer's, doesn't participate)—assert that Daniel has done right to put Leanne's mind at ease. He has acted honorably as a husband.

Daniel agrees with the men.

"It's sad," Linda says, shaking her head. Daniel agrees with this, too. But he feels he needed to honor his marriage and recognize that Leanne has supported him, in many ways, for thirty-five years now.

The discussion moves on. Daniel speaks of two "wonderful things" Leanne did recently. Her birthday came while she was in the hospital. She had called Daniel the day before and asked him to order thirty-five cupcakes from Stop & Shop. Please pick them up, she said, and bring them to her. "So I did," Daniel says. "I had some trouble, but I got help." A staff person at the hospital, he says, lent him a cart. He wheeled the cupcakes to the fifth floor. Leanne presented a treat to each patient on her ward.

A few days later, after Leanne had gotten home from the hospital, "a very large package was delivered to our door. It was so heavy we could hardly get it in," Daniel tells everyone. "But we did, and we opened it. It was a wonderful atlas. For me," from Leanne. "It was my Christmas present." Daniel has always loved maps. "So this was a fabulous gift." He pauses. "She's a very decent woman. She's just so ill and so uncomfortable with all these ailments, which the doctors can't do anything about."

. . .

In early December, Liz and I visit Joe at the veterans home. We find him in his room and climb stairs with him to the rec room—a large, bright institutional space. An enormous television airs the news. A group of residents in wheelchairs eat at a table. Finches chirp in a large cage along a far wall. A basketball arcade game stands along another. Gray sky shows through big picture windows.

"We had some snow flurries today." Joe will say this several times in the next hour. He is wearing jeans, a green polo shirt, tattered running shoes. He leads me to the corner where his models are displayed, a collection of airplanes, cars, a tractor-trailer, and a motorcycle he has built from kits. Liz has encouraged him to build things for her grandchildren, Joe's step-grandchildren. The kits let him safely use some of the skills he once used professionally, and that still form who he is. Making things for children, Liz says, helps him feel purposeful. Indeed, exercising well-instilled skills can help a person with dementia stay happy and engaged. A musician might sing long after she stops speaking. A former plumber's hands may still know how to fit pipe together. Joe, the former carpenter, shows me his built models.

Recently he has branched out; he has been assembling a pair of simple moccasins, also from a kit; he holds one up for me to see. He seems at ease here, and proprietary; he's found comfortable territory. He lays a hand on the shoulder of a man who sits at a table in a wheelchair, also sewing a moccasin. "Here's Sam," Joe says. Sam lifts rheumy eyes, glances at us, nods hello, and turns back to his stitching.

I admire a painting on an easel, a skilled and interesting portrait of a family. "That's one of Jacob's," Liz says, speaking of Joe's best friend here. Jacob has been a painter all his life. Jacob walks into the room as if on cue. He has a gentle countenance, a bald head, and big, round glasses. Jacob says he has been working off a photo that a staff person gave him. The photo—of a smiling trio—is taped to the easel. Propped up among Joe's completed car and truck models is another of Jacob's paintings, this one of Joe standing on the wing of the plane he once co-owned and flew—also done from a photograph.

Liz, Joe, and I head downstairs to the unoccupied lobby—Liz and Joe sit on a small love seat, I in an armchair by them. A Christmas tree blinks in a corner, the lights flashing off tinsel and ornaments. Staff have strung colored bulbs along the windowsills. Across the room, American and armed-services flags stand in holders. Liz, Joe, and I will spend an hour here, trying to make conversation. Joe takes Liz's right hand in his left and pulls it over to his thigh. Her lips purse. Joe will repeat a handful of stories several times during the hour. "I'm getting my hair cut this afternoon," he says. "I went down yesterday, but there were three guys in front of me." Liz looks at me knowingly. He has reported on this development twice.

Joe's confusion does seem worse. Liz's aversion to visiting him has strengthened, too. The repeated stories, his clinging to and playing with her hand—she finds these more and more trying.

She tells Joe about last night's football game.

"Just the one field goal, huh?" Joe asks.

"Yup. They're first place in their division now."

"That's good. Yeah, if I don't get down to the dayroom early enough and get it on that channel, I won't be able to see it."

"This was last night they played."

They speak more about football, about the length of quarterback Tom Brady's hair. A long pause comes around. Joe says, "I talked to Keith last night. They were out hunting. It wasn't productive, but I'm sure they had a good time." It's another of the stories that Joe has cycling in his mind. He never remembers that he's told it and is fated to repeat it.

"Yes," Liz says. "I'm sure they had good food, too."

"Oh, yes. They always have good food."

Joe says he still has the "horns" from a deer in the shed at home.

"You do?" Liz makes a face of mild disgust.

"Yeah, nailed up above the shelf to the right." Joe lifts his right hand and shows an imaginary wall. He sighs, letting his hand fall. "But the boys had a good time, I guess."

A little while later, Joe runs his fingers distractedly over Liz's. I ask him how things are going for him here.

"Very well. Very well. I keep busy. I watch movies all the time. There's a library you can check them out of. I watch with Jacob and a couple of other guys."

"An aide makes them popcorn," Liz says.

"Oh, yeah, they treat us well. There's a refrigerator with ice cream and pastries. I try to stay away from that stuff, though."

Another pause. Since arriving on this visit, I've wanted to ask Joe a difficult question, to find out more about his awareness of his situation. I try to ask gently: "Joe, what's your understanding of why you're here?"

To my surprise, he answers immediately, as if he'd just been waiting for me to ask. "I never really analyze it. My problem just came along. Something snapped in my head. I don't have much recollection of it all."

Later, I do analyze: Joe knows he has a "problem," that he's in a place for people with "problems," that his trouble has to do with his mind. Yet, he can't remember, exactly, what the problem is. I'm struck by the blend of awareness and confusion, and at the same time by his enduring sense of self—an "I" who doesn't analyze, but who has a problem. I also sense that his story that something "snapped" implies perhaps a wrongdoing, some sense that he transgressed. Or simply tragedy: bad luck befell him. Now he's doing the best he can. He doesn't—he can't—analyze, although he knows that parsing is something he might have undertaken in the past.

Joe asks Liz, "Shall we take her"—he means me—"up to the third floor and show her where I work?" He can't remember that we were just there.

"Sure," Liz says. But we don't stand. Joe tells me he makes chimes up there and cars and birdhouses. "That's great," I say.

Another pause comes around. We have talked about Joe's service in the army, about his daughter, some more about his friend Keith, and about forms from the VA that Liz has been trying to fill out. The lobby is quiet, vacant. Liz has disconnected her hand from Joe's. He sighs. He pats Liz's knee and says, "So. What have you been up to?"

Kindness

The Sunday before Christmas, at Penny's house, Mary sits with the newspaper at the kitchen table. She leafs through it, not lingering long on any page. She seems, mostly or entirely, to be looking at the pictures. She lays the newspaper back on the kitchen table. Penny asks, "Can I see the paper, Ma?" Mary gazes at her daughter, lifts the paper off the table, and holds it in front of herself, so that Penny can, literally, *see* it.

"In my *hand,* please." Penny cocks her wrist and opens her palm. She turns to me. "See where I get it?" she asks, meaning obnoxiousness. The newspaper arrives in Penny's hand. She reads aloud Mary's horoscope; it is about using your brain to improve your lot in life. There is irony in this, and in moments following: Penny takes a small box from the lazy Susan in the middle of the table, the place where vitamins, notes, and other items of daily living reside. She pulls a deck of Healing with the Fairies oracle cards out of the box. "Time to draw our cards!" Penny says. She fans the deck out, face-sides down, and holds it out to Mary, who selects a card. Penny offers me the deck, and I draw a card as well. Penny chooses last. We turn our cards over. Penny's says "Inner Power," Mary's "Kindness," and mine "Making Music."

Penny reads Mary the words on the Kindness card, speaking deliberately, in an animated voice that communicates earnestness, fun, and irony. "'Practice *kindness* today toward yourself and other people!'" she says, chin lifted importantly toward her mother. "'Look for opportunities to be *kind*.'"

Mary chuckles. She turns and smiles at me, her face warm, and also a little distracted and confused.

"Are you listening to me?" Penny asks.

"Of course," Mary says calmly, nodding once. Penny reads another line about kindness—toward oneself. Then she says to Mary, "Okay, here's your affirmation, which you will repeat after me."

"Oh, for Pete's sake," Mary says.

"'I am kind, thoughtful, and loving,'" Penny reads.

"I am kind, thoughtful, and loving," Mary says, rolling her eyes but revealing a small smile.

"'To myself and others,'" Penny says.

"To myself and others." Mary lifts her eyes and chuckles again. "Great."

Penny reads mine. I should, the card instructs, surround myself with music.

Penny reads her own card. "'Inner *power*,'" she says.

"*You* don't need any kind of power," Mary says. "You've already got it."

Penny reads on, in an Out-Loud voice, ignoring her mother, "'It is *safe* for you to be powerful. As a spiritually minded being it's impossible for you to use or abuse your power.'" She laughs.

Time to get ready for the Sunday-morning AA meeting. Penny heads down the hall to change her clothes.

I ask Mary if she slept well.

"Yes. That's one thing I have. I do sleep well."

"That's a blessing."

Penny calls from her bedroom, "She has many blessings! And I'm one of them."

"Oh, yes," Mary says.

"You can't argue with that," Penny calls.

"I wouldn't dare." Mary shakes her head and again allows a small smile.

A few moments later, Penny, still in the bedroom, calls, "I have to dress well today! I'm *powerful*!" She strides back into the kitchen, wearing jeans; a bright red, woven South American jacket over a red shirt; and her black, slip-on mules.

A week later, at noon on Christmas Day, I visit William and Joan at the nursing home. They await their holiday dinners in the small, second-floor dining room. Joan sits in her wheelchair, wearing a black boiled-wool vest embroidered with green sprigs and cardinals, a gift from her sister, and a green shirt with evergreen sprigs, a gift from her cousin.

I lean toward Joan. "Merry Christmas," I say, and smile.

She eyes me briefly, lifts the corners of her mouth in an apparently mock smile. "Oh, yes, very. *Really*."

"Oh, I don't like that tone," William says, chuckling. He smiles at me. "She might be jealous."

But Joan is having a good day. Earlier, William says, she was more animated than usual, lifting her arms when he leaned down, and returning his hug and kiss.

A woman in the far corner of the warm room, in a wheelchair, an oxygen tube in her nose, wears a bright red turtleneck and silver balls around her neck. An artificial tree stands in a corner, heavily decorated in tinsel and balls.

I sit at Joan and William's table. He and I chat. His family will come to his house later in the day; he'll have a second Christmas dinner. He saw twenty-five or thirty wild turkeys along the road on his way over here. He marvels at the stupidity of turkeys, how they get into his fenced yard and can't get out.

The staff bring food to the other patients. William and Joan wait. A middle-aged woman spoons nourishment into the mouth of an old man with oxygen tubes in his nostrils. Another woman feeds her sister, who sits nearly unconscious in a wheelchair. The able-bodied sister is having a hard time getting food into her impaired sister's mouth.

Alma, a Latina woman with an ample, molten body and a beautiful, broad, apple-cheeked face, rests solemnly at a table across the small room. William sees me watching her. He says he wants to show me something that Alma loves. He walks off briskly—a little crookedly, but nimbly—to Joan's room and returns with a foot-high, mechanical, stuffed Chihuahua. It has enormous eyes, big, pointed ears, and wears a red sombrero and a poncho. William squeezes its foot. In a soprano voice it sings "Mamacita, dónde está Santa Claus?" and dances.

Alma glances over. Recognition enlivens her face. Her mouth turns up and her eyes brighten. She laughs, heartily and in complete silence; her shoulders and breasts, her whole self, shake with mirth, but she makes no sound.

William smiles. "If you give this toy to Alma, you might not get it back." He turns, sets the dog in front of Joan, and demonstrates how to squeeze the button on the Chihuahua's foot. Joan only lifts her arthritic fingers and caresses the fabric of the poncho. William takes Joan's hand and moves it down to the dog's paw. "Pinch it, Joan. Like you do with me." He chuckles. Her fingers move back up the leg to the poncho. William moves her hand down again and pinches the spot that says PRESS. The Chihuahua dances and sings again, and Alma looks over again and shakes and smiles. Joan stares at the little dog as it sings.

Before long, William brings another toy from Joan's room: a mechanical chipmunk, Alvin, who holds a little gift. A star inside the gift flashes gently. William sets the doll on the table in front of Joan. She reaches and pulls the doll toward her. Her expression turns affectionate; her eyebrows and cheeks lift, her eyes soften.

"You like him? Give him a kiss." William holds Alvin close to Joan's face.

The corners of Joan's mouth turn up. She pokes out her tongue, delicate and pointed, and touches it to the small, brown spot that is Alvin's nose.

William laughs. "Oh, not like that."

Joan retracts her tongue. But soon she sticks it out again, and "kisses" Alvin again, tongue-tip to nose. She smiles a clownish smile. William laughs and looks at me with what seems like both apology and amusement.

William leads me down the hall to Joan's room. He shows me the fiber-optic Christmas tree, about two feet tall, that sits on a small table along the wall opposite Joan's bed. He purchased the tree three years ago, and a second one for himself, to light at home. Under Joan's he has placed Christmas figurines: a glass snowman—it's supposed to light up, but the batteries are dead—and the Chihuahua, and a Santa snowman that's supposed to play a song, but its batteries are dead, too. On the shelf above Joan's bed sit her stuffed animals, mostly bears and dogs. There's one kitten that used to meow, but it, too, has lost its juice.

In the dining room, Joan pulls Alvin toward her again. "Hello, you. I like you and your little food." The last word she says affectionately, with vowel prolonged: *fooood*. She puts a finger to the animal's small, brown nose. She leans toward him and speaks in low, indiscernible murmurs. I think of the pets—Cuddles, Buffy, Sandy, Peanuts—whom Joan loved.

Joan seems to be dozing off. Her eyelids droop, then close. "Wake up," William says. "You're falling asleep."

Joan's head is tipped back, her mouth agape. William leans over, his face close to hers. "Wake up," he says again, with a familiar, loving brusqueness.

Her eyes snap open. She stares at William, and the corners of her mouth turn up, her cheeks lift, and her eyes twinkle. In an instant, her face has transformed from flaccid and vacant, to clownish. William shakes his head in apparent bafflement.

A few moments later Joan has fallen asleep again. Perhaps. Her face is frozen, her mouth open, eyes closed. William stands. "Wake up, Joan. You're letting flies in." He gently shakes her shoulder. She doesn't respond. I worry a little. But there's something about the way her body is still composed, the way it resists William's shaking—it's not clear that this is a truly unconscious being.

"Maybe she's fooling," William says, standing over her and watching.

Joan's eyes snap open, her gaze on the ceiling. The comical smile appears again on her face. She holds it for a moment, then lets her cheeks fall. William laughs. He sits. He doesn't seem nearly as surprised by Joan's joke as I am.

"She's *funny!*" I say to William in astonishment. He shrugs. I turn to Joan. "You're funny, Joan." She looks at me blankly, as if either she has already forgotten the moment, or she doesn't see why I find her keen sense of humor so surprising.

William fills me in on nursing-home news: Eva, the woman who last spring had offered Polish instruction to an aide, who once farmed and who knew the correct weight for slaughtering pigs, died a couple of months ago, a week shy of her hundredth birthday. Terrence, the man with the missing ear, has died, too.

George is sitting with us now. He has crusty skin and oxygen tubes in his nose. He seems to be sleeping. "George is often asleep," William says.

George opens his eyes and smiles at me. "I'm a sleeper," he says agreeably.

"Except," William says, "when he's playing cribbage. He's the champ."

George just blinks.

It's time for me to go. I lean over Joan. "Merry Christmas, Joan," I say again. Her smile seems genuine this time. She murmurs something, but I can't understand.

In the hall I turn to William. I'd like to give him a Christmas hug, but I just shake his hand. He squeezes my arm. I say I'm glad that later he'll have a big, home-cooked holiday dinner with relatives.

The previous Thursday, after the support-group meeting, Rufus, William, Daniel, and I had walked out the long path of corridors. William talked about the turkey he'd just bought for his Christmas dinner at home. He had left it thawing in his fridge.

Near the hospital's front entrance, Daniel's wife, Leanne, was sitting in a chair, waiting for Daniel. William said hello; Leanne peered up at him through her round glasses. She recognized him. She once worked as a realtor, and William had inspected two houses for her clients. "You were *the* builder in town back then," she said.

"Times change," William said, smiling. "Now I make toys."

❧ "A Good Group"

By the end of the year, the group has doubled in size: a dozen or more members show up at each meeting. With the conference table fully occupied, meetings sometimes feel nearly festive, their mood bravely contrary to the business at hand. There is a sense of both heft—"strength in numbers," solidarity—and also intimacy, familiarity, continuity. "At some point," a new member says to Ben at the start of a busy session, "if this growth continues, you're going to have to think about when it stops being functional."

"Yes," Ben replies. "We've touched upon the idea of splitting the group, or adding a new one."

"Because you only have an hour," the woman declares. "And everybody wants to speak."

Many of the new people who have arrived throughout the fall have become regulars. Linda and David are in their late eighties. Linda has a regal face, aquiline nose, arcing eyebrows. Her mannerisms are lively, her eyes puffy and tired. A perky demeanor sometimes follows from sleep deprivation. She acknowledges this; she is simply wired, not happy. Her husband, David, has midstage Alzheimer's. He sits amiably by her at the end of the table, across from Daniel and Ben. He has cornflower-blue eyes and hair as white as goose feathers.

"Is it okay if we call you Dave?" Ben asks at the first meeting the couple attends.

"That's what he goes by," Linda says. Dave nods and says, "Yuh, yuh, yuh"—with an apologetic chuckle. The group soon comes to know the mannerism. It reminds me of Joe's efforts, when I visit his facility with Liz, to show that he's keeping up. Dave seems to be strenuously, agreeably participating as best he can.

Linda introduces herself, saying, "Dave's had his problem for about ten years." She tells everyone he worked sixteen years with a railroad company, and thirty-five with a utility company. He fought in the Battle of the Bulge. "Let me see," she muses. "What else can I tell you? He loves people. He can't remember, but I help him along."

"No," Dave mumbles, his gaze on the table in front of him, "I can remember."

"Well, we all help each other around here," Ben says.

"Right, right, right," Dave says with another chuckle and nod.

"So that's about it," Linda says. "I'm his secretary; I'm his maid; I'm his bedmate; I'm his cook. Everything."

"How many years have you been married?" Ben asks.

"Sixty-four," Linda says.

In later meetings, she'll say often that she craves sleep. Dave is restless at night, has awful dreams, cries out, shakes, thrashes. Perhaps he's replaying his experiences in the war. But after awakening from a nightmare, he either doesn't remember or can't describe it. He often gets up for good at four in the morning. "He likes four o'clock." Linda reaches over and gives his arm a pat. "I don't know why." Their bedroom is on the second floor, and she worries that Dave will fall, wandering alone in the dark. She worries that he'll leave the house. She always gets up with him, no matter the hour. During the day, she tries to nap, lying in an armchair with her eyes closed, still half-vigilant. But Dave discovers her and shakes her, to assure himself she's still alive.

At these times, she opens her eyes, and he says to her, "I didn't know! Your chest didn't go in and out."

Hearing this story, Ben turns to Dave. "I think you're still tuning in to things."

"Right, right, right!" Dave nods and attempts a smile.

"We have our limitations as we age, but—"

"I want her around! I don't want to lose her!"

Everyone smiles. Penny gazes at Dave with what looks like both affection and sorrow.

"She takes good care of me," Dave says.

"That's good to hear. And I bet it's important for her to hear, too," Ben says, gesturing toward Linda for comment.

"Oh"—Linda waves such concerns away with her hand—"he tells me all the time."

At a later meeting Linda says quietly, "I do lose my patience every once in a while." She reaches over and gives Dave's forearm one of her familiar, affectionate slaps.

"Is that true, Dave?" Ben asks.

Dave chuckles and nods; it's not clear that he agrees or even understands.

"I don't want him to go away," Linda says, echoing Dave's anxiety about her dying, but referring to her own complex worry: How much longer can she possibly give care? When will she have to send Dave to the veterans home—the one where Joe lives? "The doctor said, 'A lot of times the caregiver goes first,'" Linda muses. She'd answered, "I just pray for one day. I don't know what will happen. So just one day longer."

"That's what we're combating, right here," Ben says, referring to the consequences of caregiver stress. "We don't want that to happen."

"Yeah." Linda is stalwart, poised, seems to make a practice of selflessness. "I don't really have any complaints." She smiles through her exhaustion.

Katherine had also joined the group in the fall. Her husband, Harold, has Parkinson's. For decades, he'd taught government at the college; she'd worked there as a top-level administrator. Katherine has a quiet, patrician manner, her voice dry, slightly growly. She's exceptionally active for her seventy-six years. Her age is "just a number," she says. She and Harold live in a pretty white house on a wooded hillside a few miles out from the town center.

Until recently, Harold's disease had affected their lives only a little. Now his difficulties with balance and muscle tremors have Katherine picking up the slack, and feeling the strain. She is not naturally suited to caregiving, she says, to having someone depend on her. She and Harold have always pursued independent interests. She was happy, this fall, to learn that their long-term-care insurance would cover much of the cost of hiring a home health aide at night—so that Katherine could finally get some sleep.

Throughout the fall, she attended the group regularly, even though she'd never expected to join a support group. She has never seen a psychotherapist either, she says, but "I find this an extremely useful way to spend an hour." At a meeting in December, her turn comes around and she says, "Am I on?" She chuckles. Turning serious, she says she thinks Harold is showing signs of dementia. She came home one evening last week and found him standing in the dark living room. He had awakened from a nap, confused and frightened, didn't know what time it was, and Katherine was gone. On another day, he'd put the keys to his visiting son's rental car in his pocket and forgotten they were there. Katherine, her son, her son's wife—and Harold—had searched frantically for the keys. "The whole house got turned upside down," Katherine says.

Ben asks if Harold sees a neurologist.

Every four months, Katherine says. Meanwhile, she knows that "parkinsonism varies enormously. There are probably ten people we know in town at one stage or another, and they're all different." There's no way to know exactly what to expect.

Ben nods. "Well, thanks for being our newest member. Who stayed!"

"Yes, well, I'm hooked."

· · ·

A woman named Carolyn arrives in late December, at the final meeting of 2010. Her mother, Rachel, has memory loss and lives at an assisted-living facility across the river. Rachel gets her meals there and enjoys the group activities. Carolyn does her mother's laundry, manages Rachel's medical care and finances, and takes her out to dine and shop about once a week. Carolyn considers herself lucky because Rachel is exceptionally sweet, well loved at her facility, and seems happy. Yet, Rachel's easy nature has become an unexpected burden: Carolyn feels guilty for resenting her lovely mother's needs. Carolyn finds difficult, too, Rachel's obliviousness of her impairments; she doesn't recognize that Carolyn is helping her. ("And why," Rachel cheerfully asks Carolyn, "is it you go to a *caregivers* support group?") Carolyn has troublesome siblings. They come to town to "help," stay with Carolyn, and then demand Carolyn's assistance with their helping. (A sister offers to do their mother's laundry, for example, but can't find a Laundromat.) Meanwhile, over the phone, from afar, Carolyn's sisters question Carolyn's decisions about their mother's care.

Carolyn says she's trying to learn to set limits on unhelpful people. She says she needs to find ways to manage her stress—she's just not sure if that means coming to this group or, who knows, going out dancing.

Katherine says, in her reserved-yet-caring manner, "Going dancing would be fun—but this group is important. It really is." Katherine pauses. "Also, we do laugh a lot. Even at a lot of things that aren't funny."

"We *make* them funny," Ben says.

Carolyn nods and smiles. Even this one meeting, she says, "has been very worthwhile for me. I want to thank you all and wish you a happy New Year."

• • •

Penny brings Mary to the meeting at the end of the year, too—
Mary's first visit. Mary sits good-naturedly, distractedly, at the
head of the table.

"Mary, it's good to have you here," Ben says.

"I'm only here because of my daughter." Mary seems a little
nervous, as if not sure what to expect.

"Did she force you to come?"

"No, I just—"

"I'm kidding."

"She does force me to do a lot of things," Mary says, her demeanor
relaxing. "This is not one of them. I came to keep her company. I don't
know anything about this. But, I'm interested, and I'm listening."

Ben says, "It's wonderful to have the people who are being
cared for in the group sometimes."

"Well, she's caring for *me*."

"I know!" Ben smiles.

Penny laughs.

"It's an important part of the perspective, to get your side of
the story," Ben says.

"She's doing a good job."

"Yeah?"

Penny tips her head back and laughs again.

"Most of the time." Mary smiles.

"Was that a twenty-dollar bill I saw passed?" Ben asks.

The group chuckles.

"That's great," Ben says. "Could you give us two examples of
what Penny does?"

"She listens to me. That's a lot. Because I have a big mouth."

"So now you know where I get it," Penny says to everyone.

"So she listens," Ben says. "That's one. What else?"

"She takes good care of me. She makes good meals. She's a
good cook."

Penny cackles. "I love this." She turns to Ben. "Thank you. I should be slipping *you* a twenty, Ben."

Ben suggests to Daniel that Daniel might be feeling hostage to Leanne's suicidal impulses. "It's entirely possible that she will make another attempt," Daniel says. "She's very uncomfortable physically, mentally. She's in pain; nothing seems to help her, no amount of painkillers." He and Leanne hope that a new specialist at Yale can help.

Ben asks about Leanne's own interests. "Is she doing her research still?"

"Lately less so, but some."

"Is she getting to the drive-through?" Ben knows that Leanne's forays in the car to get breakfast represent a degree of independence and initiative.

"Less so. One problem is that she can't go outside." Leanne has been receiving visiting-nurse services, and according to insurance regulations, Leanne qualifies for these only if she's "homebound." So, Daniel says, "she *can* drive to Wendy's and get fast food, which she loves. But other than that, she can't go out without risking the loss of these visiting nurses." This insurance rule discourages healthy, active behavior in times of transition.

Meanwhile, Daniel says, a psychotherapist recently told Leanne that Daniel, by corresponding with his platonic, female friend, had transgressed in his marriage. "Old men," the therapist had said, "do silly things." Daniel shakes his head. The group gasps sympathetically.

. . .

Liz, who hasn't attended in a few weeks, joyfully announces the birth of her granddaughter. The group applauds.

She also reports, "Joe is now a hoarder." One day the prior week, when she'd arrived to visit him, he had said, "I had a great day today."

"Oh? What did you do?" she asked.

"I found a wallet in the bathroom with no name in it and nine dollars in there."

"Well, what did you do with it?"

"I took the nine dollars and put it in my own wallet!" he said. Everyone laughs.

Liz asked Joe, "Well, where's the other wallet now?"

"In a drawer."

"Well, you really should give that back. Give it to a nurse."

"No! There's no name in it, so it's mine."

Liz tells the group that Joe would never have behaved this way before. She asked a staff person for help. A nurse's aide said, "Oh, things like that happen all the time here." She came with Liz into Joe's room and asked for the wallet. Joe gave it to her. Liz whispered to the aide, "There was money in there."

So the aide said, "Joe, I think there were eighteen dollars in there." Joe said, "No, no, there weren't." The aide returned to the nurses' station. Liz says she turned to her husband and said, *"Joe."*

Liz rolls her eyes, imitating Joe's reaction at the time: "It wasn't *eighteen*! It was *nine*!"

The group laughs some more.

"I said, 'Well, it doesn't matter if it was nine or a hundred. It's not your money.'" Joe soon took the hoarded money to the nurses' station and slammed it onto the counter. The aide said, "Oh, thank you, Joe! That's really good of you. Thank you so much."

Meanwhile, Liz tells everyone, she continues to have trouble with the staff at the facility. A few weeks earlier, interested, like me, in how much Joe understood of his situation, Liz had asked him if he knew what his diagnosis was. He hadn't. Later Liz had reported this to the nurse-manager on Joe's floor. The nurse had expressed outrage, apparently considering the question deeply insensitive, disrespectful.

"She really laid into me," Liz tells the group. "She yelled at me like I was a twelve-year-old. She made me feel really stupid: *'Why would you ever ask him what his diagnosis is?'*"

"Well, number one, I'm his wife," Liz remembers saying.

Sarah asks, "Why would she ever *speak* to you that way?"

"Exactly." The nurse seems to Liz worn-out, jaded. "She's going to retire next August." As other staff have, the nurse also seemed to imply that Joe should not be institutionalized at all, and to blame Liz for his confinement.

The nurse said to Liz, "If Joe ever comes to anyone here and says, 'I do not have dementia, and I'm fine'—he's going home!"

"Oh, my God," Penny says.

"I said, 'You're going to send a man home who threatened my life? Not once, but twice?'"

"Did you get [what she said] in your notebook?" Ben asks.

"I have it all written down."

"She needs to be reported," Penny says. "That is unacceptable. She was having a bad day, that woman."

At five o'clock the group walks out together, past the food-service offices, right at the elevators, past mammography, into the art-display hallway. It is unusual for them to leave the meeting together; usually they drift out in small groups. Up front, Daniel sets the slow pace. No one seems to mind. Two or three abreast, they take a step at a time, shoulder to shoulder, heads bowed, chatting softly. Karen's husband, Don, who has dementia, walks next to me and says, "You could write a soap opera about Daniel's life!

Such a nice guy. But what a hard time. Boy, it makes you think you've got it easy."

I soon find myself beside Sarah, who says to me, "This is such a good group! Isn't this a good group?"

"Yes. What do *you* like about it?"

She thinks for a moment. "It has a lot to do with Ben. He makes it seem okay to say stuff you might not otherwise say."

"A kind of safety?"

"Yes, yes. Safety."

The group ambles on, spreading out through the wide, bright lobby. By the entrance and its glass doors, Sarah turns to Daniel. "Daniel, can I walk you to your car?"

"Yes, thank you." Daniel nods and tips his cap. Sarah holds the door. Daniel steps through. It has been a bright winter sunset, and even this late in the year a little light is still left in the sky.

PART V

ANOTHER YEAR UNFOLDS

🌿 Falls

The first snow of 2011 arrives in early January, and for weeks the storms keep coming. Snowblowers carve white, crystalline walls several feet high along sidewalks. On sunny days, the houses sparkle in thick, white blankets. The fire chief sends out a robo-call: Clear the snow from your roofs, he implores, so they don't cave in. The surfaces of many town roads stay packed with ice and snow.

Back in the late fall and through the end of the year, group members shared difficult struggles that, nevertheless, kept fairly stable: Penny endured frustrations in managing home health aides. Daniel's marriage swung through tolerable ups and downs, concurrent with Leanne's mood swings. Liz decided to have Joe home for Christmas and worried about having him in her house, but the visit went fine. Situations changed little. At that last meeting of 2010, Katherine had even said drily, of herself and Harold, "As a general statement, every week is pretty much like every other week. We just keep going along."

January changes that. A week after she says this, Katherine, Harold, and another couple go out to dinner, at a place downtown in an old rail station. Because Harold's disease has weakened his muscle control—including his swallowing—Harold's doctor has asked Harold several times if he can cut his food. Harold has always insisted that he can. Tonight, though, after Harold orders a steak, he agrees, reluctantly, to let Katherine cut it. His Parkinson's is worsening.

Katherine cuts only part of the meat, thinking Harold won't want more. He eats what she's sliced, then cuts more for himself. He forks one of these pieces—too big, Katherine will later say— and puts it in his mouth. He can't chew it well nor fully swallow the steak. It ends up in his windpipe. He can't cough it up.

"Are you all right?" Katherine asks. He struggles. He shakes his head and clutches his throat. Harold's effort to breathe lodges the steak deeper. Katherine tries the Heimlich maneuver, to no avail. She asks her friend if he knows how. No, he says, but he tries anyway.

The restaurant has little business that night—fortunately, Katherine will say later. The foursome are alone in the dining room. The waitstaff rush over. Someone calls 911. From that point on events go fast.

Harold loses consciousness. EMTs arrive and remove the steak from Harold's throat. But for several minutes, Harold's heart—a muscle also compromised by Parkinson's—has lacked oxygen. It has stopped beating. The EMTs can't restart it.

Harold was eighty-three. He and Katherine had been married for fifty-four years.

Not long after this, everything changes for Daniel, too. On a Tuesday in the second week of January, he drives Leanne to her psychiatrist appointment. Afterward, he helps her into the passenger seat of their small sedan. Using his cane, he walks around toward the driver's side. The parking lot is well plowed, but his foot catches on a bulge in the pavement. He goes down hard. He lies on the cold ground, stunned and in pain. He can't get up. Above him a few people gather. A couple of Good Samaritans crouch and reassure him. An ambulance arrives. EMTs hoist Daniel. At the hospital, X-rays show a broken hip. Daniel is admitted for surgery.

One in three adults aged sixty-five or older falls each year, according to the CDC. Two million of these people go to emergency rooms. Falls are the leading cause of injury among the elderly, and of death by injury, and of hospital admissions for trauma. The elderly who fall have poor balance, weak muscles, are experiencing medication side effects, or have foot problems that cause walking trouble. The prevention measures are not surprising: exercise and physical therapy to improve strength and balance; installing grab bars and other aids in seniors' homes; removing rugs, ottomans, coffee tables that can cause tripping; and adjusting medications that cause dizziness, sleepiness, or poor balance.

I wonder to myself, Did Daniel break his hip because he was struggling to help someone else at a time in life when he himself was vulnerable? Had Leanne been healthy, she would likely have been the one making sure *he* got safely into the car. Daniel's new troubles seem to stem in part from his difficult situation, his caregiving. Daniel becomes entirely dependent.

A few days after his surgery, I find him sitting in a big hospital chair by his bed. He's pale. His johnny keeps slipping off his shoulder. Daniel says he's fine, that everyone here treats him well. He misses his music, though. Later I bring him a small CD player, along with a few of my CDs, including some Brahms. Daniel will tell me later that he doesn't much care for Brahms. He finds Brahms, "please excuse the word, 'constipated.'" He means self-conscious, too restrained. Beethoven, on the other hand—so energetic, vital! Still, he thanks me graciously for the CDs.

Leanne visits Daniel in the hospital, once. She drives herself to the valet entrance, and an attendant pushes her in a wheelchair to Daniel's room. Later, kindly, she calls the local public-radio station and asks the announcer to play a recording of a Mahler symphony conducted by Gustavo Dudamel, whom Daniel admires. Leanne once nicknamed Dudamel "the Dude," to Daniel's amusement. The announcer plays the piece, and Leanne tells Daniel later that she had listened at home. But Daniel was not in his room when it aired.

Katherine comes back to the group in late January. The weeks since Harold's death have been awful—with quick preparations for a Jewish funeral and all the paperwork that comes with a spouse's demise. She tells everyone that she's glad she was spared the worst of caring for someone in a long and difficult illness. Several years before, a friend had died "of a massive coronary, after having been diagnosed with Parkinson's disease." Another friend had said of this death, "At least he was spared the indignity of continuing to live with Parkinson's." Katherine says she feels the same way about Harold's passing. "Because I hear the stories, and I've seen" life with the disease. "It's not an easy life. So I consider myself fortunate. I consider *him* fortunate."

She turns and looks around the table. "I wanted to thank you all—for the practical information, and for the moral courage. It was very helpful to have had this group."

"My condolences, Katherine," Inga says. "My father-in-law died of Parkinson's."

Carolyn, too, offers sympathy. "My stepmother, who I was very close to, died of Parkinson's ten years ago."

Katherine thanks everyone again. She says she plans to return to the group occasionally, at least for a while.

Ten days after his fall, Daniel moves to a nursing home for rehab. Over the following several days, I try to reach him there. I call the number Ben had given me for Daniel's unit. But the phone has rung on and on, or a staff person has answered and told me that Daniel is in therapy. There's only one cordless phone for the entire unit, and Daniel's cell phone is at his house. On a Thursday in late January, I begin reading his book on Gustav Mahler. In it Daniel portrays Mahler, as he has in conversation with me, as a man between cultures, at the margins of national and religious communities. I've known that Daniel believes he, too, lives on the margins, at the edge of a fast-moving, modern American world. Reading Daniel's scholarly analysis, I speculate anew that Daniel may value the support group, in part, because he feels, there, a sense of inclusion.

That afternoon, I try calling him again, before heading to the support-group meeting. An unfamiliar male voice answers the phone.

"I'm trying to reach Daniel Biel."

I hear the man turn and ask Daniel if he wants to take a call.

Next I hear Daniel's voice: "Hu-llo?"

"Hi, Daniel."

"Hi, Nell," Daniel says, his voice falling into a flatter tone than usual.

"It's not easy to reach you there."

"Yes, I've heard that," he says. "There are no phones in the rooms."

"That's too bad. Daniel, I'm just calling to check in and say hello before I go off to the group."

"Thank you." He pauses. "Nell, I have some very, very sad news."

"Oh?" I say.

"Leanne has died," he says. "She killed herself."

🌿 A Sense of Purpose

No one in the group has heard about Leanne, including Ben. I reach him on his cell phone. Daniel has asked me to tell no one yet but Ben, who is both stunned and not surprised. He had long been concerned about Leanne. Back in March, at a meeting that only Penny, William, and Rufus had attended, Ben had brought up the issue of suicide. He seemed to want simply to register that he was concerned. Over the hour, the conversation had waxed philosophical and reflective. Ben said that on his psychiatric ward he had seen people admitted as suicidal and later diagnosed with cancer. Soon "they were scrabbling hard to try to survive the cancer. It rules out that suicide is always about wanting to die. Usually it's more about wanting to stop the pain, the psychological pain."

Leanne had died in her bed, Daniel will later add. She had again taken an overdose of her medications. She had left three photographs on the kitchen table, a "kind of shrine": a portrait of her sister, who'd committed suicide, also by an overdose of medication, twenty years earlier; and one each of her father and mother, both also gone for years. Still in the nursing home, Daniel had learned about the photos from a friend. He sees the shrine as, in part, a rebuke to him—an admonishment, perhaps, for his failure as a husband, his failure to love Leanne well enough, care enough about her, and as well as her original family did. She had left no note.

Leanne had often said that once Daniel was "gone," she wouldn't stick around. He hadn't died, but perhaps she had experienced a similar void—the pointlessness of an empty house, her great physical and mental pain. She had been living alone for two weeks—with only the help, for a few hours each day, of the woman they'd hired as an aide. As Ben had presaged months before, Leanne must have sought to escape psychological pain. Ben had also said, back in March, that being able "to muster and access resources" protects people from self-harm—as could having a sense of connection to something larger. "Evaporation of purpose is a good sign that somebody's at risk." For Leanne, perhaps it was also a flight from feeling abandoned. Who knows; as I learned with my grandmother, suicides take their reasons away with them.

My grandmother, also, fled psychological pain: the fear of a dismal, dependent future. She refused both "care," the tending of family, and "cure," the often-frightening world of medicine. Surely no one could have cared for Leanne in a way that would heal her. With almost no one to tend her at all, Leanne opted out. Hildegard and Leanne fled psychological suffering, each in her way—and in the case of my grandmother, an anticipated future of suffering—through a final, forceful act of will.

The day after Daniel tells me about Leanne's death, I drive to his "nursing and rehabilitation center." The low-slung brick building is bordered to the south by a Home Depot and elsewhere by snow-covered farm fields. The facility's white columns and ornate faux balconies seem meant, as with so many similar facilities, to make it less generic and institutional, which they don't. In a lobby, two orange tabby cats lounge in armchairs. But down the institutional hall, the scene, by now so familiar to me, seems glum: a collection of white-haired, shrunken people hunched in wheelchairs, many with their eyes closed and mouths open. A young man stands among them, hugging a ball, ready to lead an exercise class, if anyone's ready to follow.

Clutching a fistful of purple tulips, I ride an elevator to the second floor. I find Daniel tended by three friends from his academic life—a husband and wife and another woman. They've brought him his mail from home and are helping him organize his belongings, compiling the phone numbers he's written on scraps of paper and strewn on his bedside table. One of the women has brought a few of Leanne's clothes from Daniel's house so that Daniel can pass them along to the funeral director, who will stop by.

The friends leave. I sit by Daniel's bed. He's wearing his usual worn corduroys and a charcoal-gray, V-neck sweater. On top of the professorial sweater, someone has helped him pull on a heavy, gray sweatshirt with faux-sheepskin lining. It's a workingman's sweatshirt and looks out of place. He'd complained of being cold, and a staff member had brought it to him, out of a collection of clothing left behind by others.

He looks thinner; he says he *has* lost a little weight. The food, he says, is awful.

We talk a little about Leanne and chat mostly about his experience in the nursing home. For the next two months, he will live here, work toward walking again, and cope with his sudden and traumatic loss. He praises the physical-therapy staff. They work him hard, he says, and the exercises are often painful. But he's proud of his progress. His surgeon tells him that the hip X-rays look good and show he's healing well. Both the doctor and the physical therapists insist that Daniel *will* get back on his feet—although he'll need a walker.

Daniel tells a physical therapist of his love for Mahler. The therapists often try to get him to talk, to distract him during the difficult exercises. "She probably had never heard of Mahler," he tells me later. So he is stunned when, the following week, the same therapist says she has a surprise for him. She places a CD into a player, and from the speakers he hears the adagietto from the fourth movement of Mahler's Fifth Symphony. Hearing his beloved music, Daniel weeps at the therapist's kindness.

He will tell me later that he doesn't listen to Mahler's music as much as he used to "because of its extreme melancholy. At my age, it's not so appealing" as it used to be. When you're young, melancholy may be romantic, meaningful; when you're old, perhaps, it is overwhelming.

Daniel has been hearing regularly from members of the support group: Liz and Penny call; Inga sends a long letter; Katherine and Sarah visit. Each week, I bring flowers and food—sometimes a deli sandwich, often a single piece of fruit. He says he gets no fresh fruit from the nursing home's kitchen; but he asks me to bring only one piece at a time so that none goes to waste. He eats little.

In the afternoon on Saint Valentine's Day, I bring orange and white tulips and a clementine. In his room, leaning against the head of his bed, is a long cardboard tube wound with red ribbon and stuck with shiny hearts—a Valentine's scepter. Daniel explains that one of the staff had come to him in the morning and said, "You *have* to come to the Valentine's Day party."

"No, thank you," Daniel said. "I'd rather not."

"You have to. You're going to be king!"

Daniel had reluctantly consented. He was wheeled down to the rec room. Music was already playing. "It may have been Frank Sinatra," he says. He and another woman, the Valentine's queen, were each presented with oversize scepters and fitted with crowns. They sat side by side. A lot of people were there, Daniel says. "A few people got up and *danced*," he says with amazement. "Luckily, we didn't have to make a speech." He shakes his head.

Although the event lacked the gravitas and decorum that Daniel prefers, he seems to have gotten a small boost of energy from being feted. He's also recently found a dinner companion—a "dignified" woman, he says—a former schoolteacher who is also staying at the nursing home for rehab. He enjoys their conversations. He thinks he still has a long time to serve here, though. No one talks to him about a date for going home.

• • •

He confesses that he is only slowly getting his mind around Leanne's death.

"You're sort of in a capsule here," I suggest.

"Yes." In some ways it is good he's here, he says. "Because there are people with me." He says he often thinks of things that he wishes he could tell Leanne. Perhaps he means just the odd, mundane daily events that spouses share with each other—such as the absurdity of being dubbed Valentine's king. Who knows, maybe he and Leanne would have shared a rare, private heartwarming laugh.

He thinks it's going to take time for him to comprehend that she is gone—"probably until I get home to that empty house."

🌿 "Buddha, Saint, or Dead"

In mid-March, a beautiful day, windy and mild, the snow nearly melted, I visit Daniel again. I walk from a quickening, early-spring world into the seasonless landscape of nursing-home care, again past the bright and institutional rec room, down the colorless hall, up in the elevator. Daniel is perched on the side of his bed. It is the first time I've seen him sitting up on his own since he broke his hip. He looks nearly back to his former self.

He tells me he recently visited his house, his first time home since his injury and Leanne's death. A friend drove; an occupational and a physical therapist came along.

"The first thing I did when I got into the house," Daniel says, "was go to the CD player"—he starts to weep—"and put on Beethoven's Seventh."

I nod. "Why that piece?"

He considers for a moment, then says that he considers Beethoven the most inspiring, uplifting, of all the composers. And the Seventh Symphony is a favorite. He *needed* to hear it. "Beethoven builds me up," he says. He reminds me about the photos that Leanne had left on the kitchen table. They were still there. He tells me that when he moves home for good, he'll leave the photos on the table for a while.

"To honor her wishes?" I ask.

"Yes."

He says the PT and OT gave him good advice. He'll need grab bars on the bathtub, and he should place his most used kitchen things within reach on the counter, have someone tape or remove the area rugs, always keep the phone near him, and always wear his medical-alert button. He must replace the wheeled desk chair that has no armrests—it's too dangerous—and use a sturdier one instead.

I imagine Daniel nodding dutifully at each suggestion. "Okay," he would have said—eternally a student in prewar German schools.

After the visit, his friends took him out for lunch in a diner. Daniel ate a grilled-cheese sandwich with sliced tomato, french fries, and minestrone soup. It felt good to be out of the facility, he recounts to me, eating food that pleased him.

Today, though, he seems weary and sad. He's eager to get out for good, but anxious about returning home alone and coping.

I suggest that he's been through trauma.

"Yes." He nods slowly. "I'm just worn down from coping with all of these—circumstances. And I'm so old."

A week later, a friend drives Daniel home to stay. Daniel steps into his pleasant, empty kitchen—tidy, with a green-checked linoleum floor, Formica counters, wood cabinets, a small wooden table. The kitchen window looks out on white pines. The friend unloads bottles of medicines, boxes of painkillers, and paperwork onto the kitchen table, by the photos that Leanne had left. In the living room, Daniel finds his familiar navy-blue couch, the tall-backed desk chair that Leanne sat in—and beyond, the bright picture window overlooking his quiet street.

He begins settling into life alone.

The following Thursday, I help him into his car, fold his walker and put it in the trunk, and drive him across the river to the hospital. I pull up at valet parking, help him out of the car, unfold his walker, and place it in front of him. I'm learning how to perform caregiving tasks. Some are familiar—I knew these from tending my young children. But there are new skills, too. A walker is different from a stroller; so is a wheelchair. And I must treat Daniel as an adult, despite his dependence. At the hospital's entrance, the valet looks past Daniel and asks me, "Do you want me to take him inside while you park the car?" The young man seems to interpret the scene—a middle-aged woman helping an old man—and assume the old man's inability to make decisions. The valet interprets dependence as incompetence.

I turn to Daniel. "What do *you* want?"

Meanwhile, Mary and Penny have been making their ways together onward through slow decline. A few weeks before, Penny, Inga, and I met, as usual, for lunch and conversation. I asked Penny a question having to do with Medicaid's five-year "lookback" into an applicant's finances. Penny looked at me and said incredulously, "If my mother is *alive* in five years?" She paused. "If my mother is alive in five years, I'm either going to be dead, or a *buddha*." She rephrased ecumenically, "I'm either going to be dead, or a *saint*."

This day that I bring Daniel back to the support group is also Mary's birthday. Penny will be bringing Mary to the meeting. I roll Daniel, in a hospital wheelchair, along the corridors, to his usual spot at the conference-room table.

"Daniel!" Karen says from up the table. "Welcome back."

Don gives a warm hello. Daniel smiles and nods.

My cell phone rings. It's Penny, calling from the road. She asks me to let Ben know she'll be late. She doesn't know how she'll drop off her mom, park the car—

I say I'll walk back out and pick up Mary at the entrance.

"That would be great," Penny says.

Out front, Mary gives me her usual warm hello—but doesn't remember me. We set off down the long lobby, Mary hustling along with her walker.

"Happy birthday. It's today, right?"

"Yes." She's wearing a bright pink sweatshirt—a festive birthday color—decorated with a small fuchsia flower.

"We're going that way." I point toward the stairs at the end of the long lobby. Mary shuffles ahead and stops near the stairs. "How much *farther*?" she asks, puffing. She turns her walker and sits on its seat. Penny appears. She hands me a to-go carton of Dunkin' Donuts coffee. Mary stands. Penny points the way around the stairs and on down the corridor, and Mary walks on, puffing. At the next corner she sits again. "How much farther?" she asks again. Not far, Penny says. It's tedious, and the corridors seem endless, probably for all of us.

Inga, Penny says, is bringing cake.

In the conference room, Mary sits next to Daniel at the head of the table. Ben has arrived and has brought Daniel two pieces of apple pie, wrapped in plastic, from the coffee shop. They sit on the table in front of Daniel.

"Who wants decaf coffee?" Penny asks.

Linda asks Inga if she made the cake; it's white, has purple flowers and green leaves, and sits in a plastic case.

"No, but I'm good at buying them!" Inga says.

Penny passes out coffee and cream packets.

Carolyn, the woman who joined a few months before, walks in, and then a newcomer. William's here, and Linda and Dave, and Karen and Don, and four other regulars, and Ben. Daniel sits quietly, looking down at the table. Ben tells everyone that Sarah couldn't make it today.

The cake says *Happy Birthday, Mary!* Mary says that this is the first cake that's ever borne her name. It's possible.

Everyone sings with tuneless gusto. Mary smiles and nods, and we all applaud.

"We practiced for three months," Don says, deadpan.

"Speech!" Penny calls. Mary either ignores her or doesn't hear.

Penny grips the knife and moves it over the cake—too close for comfort, apparently, to Mary, who scowls. Penny catches the look, cuts into the cake, sees that she's sliced into Mary's name, says, "Oops!" and laughs.

The table is crowded; we sit shoulder to shoulder, chatting and sliding forks into icing. William says, "We're going to have to get a bigger room pretty soon!"

Ben's voice breaks into the chatter. "I was hoping we could start with you, Daniel."

Slowly the room goes silent. Daniel sits up. "Well, I just—I can't possibly express in words how happy I am to be back." His face is serious, though. He takes a breath. "I thank all of you most cordially for your messages, your visits, your gifts, your calls. They kept my spirits up. I'm planning to come back regularly if I possibly can."

"Good," Penny says, and everyone smiles.

"Thank you so much." Daniel gives a little bow and leans back into the wheelchair. Everyone applauds. At the opposite end of the table, Linda's husband, Dave, chuckles amiably.

That's all, Daniel says, for now.

Ben turns and asks Mary if today is her actual birthday.

She nods. "Just don't ask me how old I am."

"How old do you *feel*?" Inga asks.

"Sixteen!" Mary says.

Penny offers news of her caregiving—a recent visit to a pulmonologist, his recommended adjustments to Mary's CPAP machine. "Meanwhile, we're just going to keep celebrating this birthday as long as we can." Penny turns to her mother and sees that Mary is gesturing toward the cake—a waving motion, as if shooing a fly off its surface. "Did you want more?" Penny asks with amusement, raising her eyebrows.

"No. But if you can't talk and cut cake at the same time, then just cut cake!" Mary sighs with maternal exasperation and takes a sip of coffee. Everyone laughs.

Penny looks around the table. "Has everybody," she asks with mock primness, "had cake who wants cake?"

No one requests more.

"It's delicious," Karen says.

"You don't *have* any!" Mary says. "How can you say it's delicious?"

"Already ate it."

More laughter.

"Anyway," Penny says, her hand back on the cake knife, "everything is good" in the world of caregiving.

"Don't cut your finger," Mary says.

Penny smiles. "This is a good celebration. It's really nice to be here."

Inga says she has been enjoying work in New York and spending time with colleagues. Louise is fine enough, she says, but she won't be up to the Europe trip they had planned. Liz says she is still pulling back on her visits to Joe. She speaks to him on the phone every night, though. "It's only about a three-minute conversation. But it works for him."

Penny pushes the birthday cake toward the middle of the table, away from herself and Mary.

Mary turns to Ben. "She's making sure I don't eat too much," she says.

Ben nods amiably, a bit distractedly. "Good."

Mary pauses. She peers at Ben, pursing her lips. "Did you really mean that?"

Ben startles a little; he has, heedlessly, implied that Mary should watch what she eats. He ducks his head, looks at her from the corner of his eyes sheepishly.

Inga cackles.

"What a terrible thing to say to me," Mary says in mock exasperation.

"You're not going to throw your coffee at me, are you?" Ben asks.

Mary peers into her cup. "There's not enough here to."

"Oh, man." Penny looks at the ceiling and blows out her cheeks.

"Phew," Ben says, smiling.

"Well," Mary says, "you asked, and I answered."

"I walked right into that one, didn't I?"

"Yes, you did."

"Okay!" Ben says. "Moving on to Carolyn."

Carolyn's main struggle lately has been with her sisters. "It got so stressful for me that I reached a point where I couldn't function. I had a day where I just couldn't get off the couch."

"It's depressing," says Anne, the occasional member whose mother had mouth cancer and now copes with chronic pain.

"It's very depressing. I'd prefer to have nice relationships in the family, cordial at least." But if this isn't possible, Carolyn will prioritize "taking care of the one person in the family who really can't take care of herself, my mother," over sibling relations.

She's working on saying no to people: Her boss has requested that Carolyn work more hours. Carolyn's daughter has upped her own hours at work and will be less available to care for Rachel. "I told my daughter what I *was* willing to do. I told her, 'Absolutely not on Thursdays, because *that* is my group'"—this meeting. Carolyn smiles, makes a fist, pumps it once gently, and laughs.

Liz and Inga call, "Yes!"

"I *need* my group," Carolyn says, and nods.

Linda crosses her fingers, holds them up, and looks around the table. "I don't want to jinx myself, but it's been a good week." She's not superstitious but, still, fears that if she speaks about having had decent sleep, or an easier week, with David, that very night David will be restless and keep her up.

Ben asks David how he's doing.

"Good, good, good!" David says, nodding earnestly.

"Glad to hear. You've got on another dapper sweater today," Ben says. It's bright turquoise and shows off David's white, white hair.

"Hi, William," Ben says.

William looks around the table. Not much new to report, he says.

"How about just one image," Ben says, "of Joan over the last week."

"Sleepy at times." She's been dozing at the table more often. Also making a mess of her food. "Stuff like that. But otherwise she's—you can't expect much. She can't tell me what's wrong with her."

"What are *you* up to?"

William says he's been doing some work around the house. He made a coffee table, but he messed it up and had to start over. He chuckles. "Plus, I'm carving birds."

"I keep feeling guilty about that," Ben says—he'd told William a while ago that he wanted to learn how to whittle. So William provided Ben with wood and tools, but Ben hasn't yet found time to use them.

"I've got the sandpaper for you, too."

"Do you? Well, I'm going to be a wood-carver *some*day, William."

"It's good to be here," Katherine says. "I'm doing okay." She has just returned from ten days of skiing in British Columbia with her son and his family. She enjoyed the time away. She has been overwhelmed with the paperwork that follows a death—"the stuff that has to be done to get Harold's name off of bank accounts, and so on. It's just endless. *Endless.* Sooner or later it'll be done, but it's very hard, and stressful." While she was away, someone from a bank left a phone message that the institution would be freez-ing Katherine's checking account because Harold's name was still on the account. "I thought, *'Aaaah.'*" Katherine makes claws and waves them in the air.

"That's been resolved. But every once in a while I think, 'Why do they have to make it so hard?' I mean, it's hard anyway." She turns to Carolyn. "I wanted to tell you that I really admire your strength."

Carolyn smiles ruefully. "You mean when I was lying on the couch for a whole day?"

Katherine says she's having difficulty with her brother, her only sibling, concerning an aunt who's dying in Florida. "It's very, very troubling," she says to Carolyn, "when you have this kind of potential break with a sibling. You don't want the break, but—the reality is very hard to deal with. So I think that you're doing admirably."

"Thank you. I don't feel that." Carolyn puts a hand to her forehead.

"I could tell that you don't. But you should."

Ben asks Katherine about what she did during the ski vacation. He seems to assume that, given her age—seventy-six—Katherine stayed in the lodge.

"I skied!"

"Oooh!" the group says.

"Did she say she *skied*?" Karen calls from down the table.

Everyone laughs.

"Weren't you afraid you were going to break your hip or something?" Karen asks.

"No, no. I'm a skier. It's part of who I am."

Ben turns to Daniel. "We're back to you. Any fun stories about your adventure?"

"No." Daniel shakes his head firmly. "It wasn't fun." He pauses. "I can only repeat what I said at the beginning, that I'm tremendously grateful to all of you for your kindness. It's been overwhelming. You really sustained me with your friendship. For which I'm tremendously grateful—now especially that I'm alone."

"Could I share some things about you?" Ben asks, smiling. "I promise I won't embarrass you too much." He mentions the Saint Valentine's Day scepter.

Daniel shakes his head.

Ben turns to the group. "He was the Saint Valentine's Day king at the nursing home."

"Oooh!"

Daniel shakes his head again, but smiles a little, too.

"Did you take the scepter home with you?"

"No, I didn't. I did not want to be reminded of that place."

"That's understandable," Penny says.

"I don't think you played any bingo, did you?" Ben asks.

"No."

"You were very noble."

"I was probably a good patient. I did what they asked me to do."

"How was the food?" Linda asks.

"The food was *terrible,*" Daniel says with sudden force.

People chuckle.

"Are you keeping busy at home?" Linda asks.

Daniel seems to have warmed to the conversation. Like Katherine, he's "deluged with paperwork. Taxes are coming up; I have to work on them. It's going to be very difficult to get out from under this tremendous amount—correspondence, documents— that has piled up since this happened."

There's a pause; the heat whirs. It's five o'clock, the end of the hour. Ben looks sideways, affectionately, at Daniel. "It's so nice to have you back," Ben says. "We're going to keep you coming here."

Daniel nods, head bowed.

Ben turns to Mary. "Mary, so nice to have you. You keep being kind to your daughter."

"Oh, yes," Mary says, shaking her head.

"She'll keep being kind to you."

"Oh, yes."

Penny, sitting to Ben's and Mary's right, looks at the ceiling and says, in prayerful voice, "God, I hope so." She gazes at her mother, then glances at Ben, a look on her face that is at once beatific and amused, her chin resting in her hand.

Penny turns back to her mother. "I hope I can be kind to you."

🌿 Spring

When she first came to the group, Sarah, the psychiatric nurse, had felt angry at her husband, Walter. She had wanted to say, "Snap out of it!" By now, a year later, she says, her anger is more "global." She is furious at her whole damn situation. "I'm angry at being alone, and not alone"—not released. "You can't move on." She finds herself bitterly envious of a friend who came home one day to find her fifty-two-year-old husband dead of a stroke.

I ask Sarah if she thinks we need new rituals that acknowledge ongoing, unclear loss, as a funeral recognizes a death. She thinks she has been creating rituals inadvertently—stumbling upon meaningful acts of letting go. She sorts through Walter's clothes and relives the time in Hawaii when he wore a particular shirt and she bought a skirt to match. She places Walter's suits in a bag and takes them to a food pantry. Downscaling for a move into a smaller apartment, she gives away mementos, precious figurines, to charity, too. They are acts of generosity, prompted by loss.

The unintentional rituals of slow loss will continue for Sarah in months to come. Walter will move to the nursing home. One day Sarah will wheel him down the hall and into a common room, hoping to watch a golf tournament with him. They had always loved to play and follow golf. She will park him in front of the TV. But soon he'll grow distracted, agitated, and wheel himself away. She'll force herself not to do what she would have done before— say, "Hey! Come back here!" Instead, she'll release him, just a little—not just out of the room, but out of her life.

Every time she takes the elevator to Walter's floor and hears the doors ding and sees them slide open, "my heart is in my throat." She'll be afraid of what she'll find, what new loss. "Every time I go in, I have to meet him where he is."

In a year, in the spring of 2012, she'll take a trip by herself to Maine, check into an inn where she and Walter often vacationed. She will walk the beach alone, "a batty old lady," wearing "a long, purple granny skirt, and a butt bag, and a big yellow hat."

She'll amble along the edge of the surf, and the hem of her skirt will get soaked. She will stroll by young couples, holding hands. "Never stop holding hands!" she will call to them, smiling. To another couple she will say, "Never stop sharing ice cream!"

She will arrive home and think to herself, "You're facing the same problems. But you're a little bit healed." The trip, she'll tell me, had been another ritual of letting go.

This May of 2011 brings rain and warmth. Leaves and blooms emerge everywhere: lilacs, apple blossoms, beech, forsythia along the hospital parking lot, red tulips in yards. Purple azaleas blossom along the college's pond.

One soft, misty evening, Mary and Penny sit eating dinner—chicken and sautéed zucchini and baguette—at the kitchen table. *All Things Considered* murmurs from the boom box on a nearby shelf.

Mary looks at her plate. "I'm done with this," she says, apparently expecting action. Penny stands, clears dishes to the sink, and brings Mary a bowl of Jell-O. Penny squirts whipped cream on top. She sits. In front of her, on the lazy Susan, sits a page-a-day calendar of Dalai Lama quotes. Today's page reads, *For as long as space endures, and for as long as living beings remain, until then may I, too, abide to dispel the misery of the world.*

Penny sees me reading the quote and says of the calendar in

general, "That's helpful." Pause. "Not!" She laughs. "It's supposed to help you be calm, peaceful, and mindful."

From a plastic pitcher, she pours me iced decaf mixed with Lactaid and stevia.

Mary takes a bite of Jell-O. "I haven't heard from Sophie in a while."

Penny pauses ever so briefly, her demeanor calm. "I think she called *yesterday*." She looks at her mother.

"Uh," Mary grunts. "How could I forget so quick?"

"That's just what you do," Penny says cheerfully—kindly. "You have a built-in forgetter."

Mary grunts again.

Outside, Penny's garden is exploding with new growth. A few weeks later, Penny picks an armload of flowers from her garden, carries it inside, and piles the blooms on the kitchen counter. She pulls a vase from a cabinet and draws sprigs from the pile—white feverfew, apricot foxglove, purple lupine, yellow snapdragon. She creates a lacy wedge. She threads long, feathery *Itea* in among the other blooms. The *Itea* curve out from the wedge like swans' necks. Penny lifts the bouquet, carries it to the chest behind the couch where her mother sits. Mary stares at the television with placid eyes. Penny's flowers arc over Mary, as if crowning her beloved head.

Exodus

In September, the day comes that Penny has dreaded and hoped for, worried about and planned toward—the day she'd long tried to predict. On a warm, damp Saturday morning, I arrive at Penny's house and find her brothers and sisters already gathered in the kitchen. As AA urges its followers to do, the siblings have "shown up." They'll help meet their mother's—and sister's—needs. Angie, the home health aide, has come, too, and a friend of Penny's named Jennifer. Mary sits in her office chair at the kitchen table. Penny's brother Jim is perched on the seat of Mary's walker, looking jovial. Penny introduces me.

"Hu-llo, Nell," Jim says languidly in a mock-Irish accent.

Penny's eyes are puffy and red—sad. But whatever sorrow had happened earlier, now she scurries in and out of rooms, organizing and packing. Seeming to recognize in Penny an earned authority, the siblings follow her lead. So do I. Journalist-cum-caregiver, I follow Penny down the hall and into Mary's bedroom. She issues instructions. Using permanent markers, Jennifer and I label clothes with Mary's initials and her soon-to-be room number. Jim unscrews a mirror from one of Mary's two dressers. He packs knickknacks into a box.

Mary's material life, once pared by her move to this house, is trimmed further.

Back in the kitchen, labeling done, I sit at the table with Jennifer and Mary. Jim and Steve tromp back and forth through the kitchen: a mattress glides by, then a box spring. Sophie makes a fresh pot of coffee. Mary requests decaf. The scent of hazelnut fills the room. Jim warbles and whistles as he travels back and forth between driveway and bedroom. The siblings unearth history: Sophie finds their father's old coin collection. Deborah brings Mary a photo of Jim from 1973, hair down to his shoulders, with a prom date.

"Who is that?" Mary asks of the girl.

"Phoebe Danvers," Deborah says.

"Ooh, yes." Mary repeats the name. Perhaps she remembers. She sips her coffee. She says to nobody in particular, as Jim and Steve traipse through with her dresser, "I don't know *what* they're doing."

"It's okay," Penny says, pausing in the kitchen. "It'll all make sense soon."

"I'm not worried." Mary shrugs. "You guys know what you're doing." She seems to rest in the comforting bustle of her focused children.

The siblings sing and banter. Deborah says, walking through the living room, "Are we the loud family—or what?"

"Where are they *going* with all that stuff?" Mary asks.

"They're putting it in the car for your new apartment," Angie, the home health aide, says.

Mary watches, considering, perhaps making sense of it all for just that moment. "Oh my gosh, there's so much stuff. I don't know where they're going to put it all."

Jim comes into the kitchen from the hall with a package of Depend for Women. He displays it, Vanna White–style, eyebrows raised, sliding sideways through the living room. "I didn't know you wear those, Jim," Jennifer says wryly.

Penny has moved in and out of rooms, supervising. In the kitchen, she asks, looking mostly at Jennifer, "So do you think this house would be good for a party?" She's thinking toward her new life.

Yeah, Jennifer and Angie both say, sipping their coffees.

"Can I come?" Mary asks.

"Oh, of course!" Penny says, and heads back down the hall.

An injury had tipped the scales, spurring Penny to fill out application forms. She had been moving her car out of the garage and—long story short—the car had rolled over her foot. She'd had to stay home for several days. Mary kept asking Penny what was wrong: Why was Penny home? Mary couldn't remember from one moment to the next what had happened. Penny realized that she still expected her mother to recall details that mattered. She fretted about what would have happened to her mother had Penny gotten *seriously* hurt. Her injury, for whatever complex reasons, triggered Penny to act.

Three weeks before Mary's move, a Tuesday morning, Sally, the nurse-manager of Mary's future home, arrived at Penny's door. Sally was middle-aged, wore a name tag from her facility, carried files, had neatly coiffed, chin-length hair and manicured nails. Penny invited her to sit at the kitchen table. Mary came down the hall with her usual force and lowered herself into her office chair. Angie, the home health aide—African-American, with thin, muscular arms and short, spiky hair—puttered around, taking out trash, wiping counters. Occasionally she'd interject comments as Sally interviewed Mary.

The administrator peered over half-glasses. "I understand you're interested in looking at an apartment at Allen Manor," she said to Mary. "Is that right?"

"I don't know," Mary said a bit peevishly. She pursed her lips. "Am I?"

"Yes," Penny said to Sally. "We've talked about this many times."

Sally began reading through a list of standard questions, with no apparent logic to their order: Which hospital, Sally asked, would Mary want to go to should there be an emergency?

Penny named one.

Which "services" did Mary "receive" from Penny? Did Mary receive help with "activities of daily living"? The nurse-manager called these ADLs. She asked if Angie helped with ADLs, too.

Yes, Angie said. "And if I'm slow, she does it herself!"

"So it's shower-with-assist?" Sally asked.

"Assistance is because of the fall risk," Penny interjected flatly. Penny hoped that Sally wouldn't decide that Mary was too impaired for assisted living—that a nursing home was required. Problems that would disqualify Mary included high fall risk, incontinence, inability to take her own medications.

"Mary, what will be your reasons for making the move?" Sally asked, apparently another of the standard questions.

"*I* don't want to go."

Penny had brought up the topic of moving before. Mary had said, "You can't *wait* to get rid of me."

"Mom," Penny had replied, "it's going to be hard at first for both of us. But they're going to love you up. And you'll see me every day. I'm going to make sure they're doing their job right."

The nurse-manager said to Mary, "There are lots of reasons people go. Support with your care, socialization." Sally paused and clarified, "Spending time with people your age."

Mary turned to her daughter. "That bothers *you,* not me," Mary said, meaning the "socialization" part.

The questions went on: Has Mary visited a doctor in the last year due to illness? Has she visited an ER in the past year? Has anyone called 911 on Mary's behalf?

No, Mary said to all.

Has Mary gained or lost weight in the last six months?

"I have no idea!" Mary said, shaking her head. "I *never* weigh myself."

"On a daily basis, your girl helps you. What do you do for yourself? Are you able to comb your hair? Get dressed?"

"I don't need *any* assistance."

"Do you use your walker all the time in your house? Are you able to get out of the chair and out of bed by yourself, able to do all your transfers?"

Mary nodded.

"In the past six months, has there been any history of falling?"

No, Mary said. (Mary had fallen a few months before. Penny said nothing to Sally now.)

Do you still drive?

Mary laughed. No. She used to, but "you wouldn't want to see me drive now!"

Around came the issue of incontinence. "Mary, do you have any trouble getting to the bathroom on time?"

"No. I wear a pad."

Penny smiled quietly. She'd heard Mary give this practical answer to doctors before.

"Are you able to manage that on your own? To change it?" Sally asked.

"Yes."

"Any problems with your bowels?"

"No."

Penny said nothing.

"Okay." Sally wrote on her form. "Now, these are some questions I *have* to ask you: What is your name?"

Mary told her.

"What month are we in?"

Mary paused, the corners of her mouth turning up. "Ooh, I don't know," she said coyly. "But I'll tell you in a minute." She picked up the newspaper that lay next to her plate and scanned the banner for a moment. "It is"—she paused—"September."

"And the year?"

"Oh, yes. It's 19—" Mary looked again at the paper. "It's 2011."

"What time of day is it, approximately?"

Mary paused. "It's morning. Close to noon." (It was ten o'clock.)

Sally asked whether Mary had a history of mental illness or addiction.

No, Mary said.

"She does take an antidepressant," Penny said.

Angie, walking by, asked, "She does?"

"That's the little, peach oval one in the morning," Penny said.

Oh, Angie said, and headed into the hall.

Penny asked Sally how medications would be given at Allen Manor.

"It's a SAMM program. Self-administration medication man-

agement." Sally addressed Mary: "It helps you stay independent." Sally explained that CNAs—certified nursing assistants—would offer the medication. Mary would have to be able to take the pills— or in the case of her eye medication, apply the drops—herself.

Standing in the kitchen, Angie asked about the ratio of CNAs to residents.

"Thirteen to one," Sally said.

Penny said, "Wow, they must be busy."

"There are ways," Sally said with apparent judiciousness, "to stagger the tasks so that the care is manageable. People take showers at different times, and so on. Mary might not want a shower every day." Sally paused, apparently looking for the right words. "In the elder population, *perspiring* is not usually an issue. Everything just kind of dries up." She smiled primly and turned back to her list.

"Mary," Sally asked, "let's say your heart stops beating. Do you want to be resuscitated? Do you have a DNR?"—an order that no one try to revive Mary should she lose consciousness.

It was a sudden shift in topic. "What's that?" Mary said, frowning.

"I believe she does," Penny said in a flat, slightly annoyed tone.

"We would need one of those on file," Sally said. "If you decide you do not want to be resuscitated. If you don't have a DNR, they will treat you like a full code." As if acknowledging that Mary might not have understood, Sally adds, "They will do everything they can to resuscitate you."

Mary showed no reaction.

Sally asked, "Have you decided on, or chosen, a funeral home?"

"We're all set with that," Penny said.

"All right," Sally said, assessing her form. She looked again at Mary. "Any questions?"

"No," Mary said gruffly.

"Have you visited Allen Manor?"

"I don't think so."

Penny explained that Mary had visited twice—once with Sophie, and once with Penny herself.

"Oh, that's right," Mary said.

Later Penny would tell me that she found Sally "cold and clinical," that the interview reminded her that assisted-living facilities are *businesses*. At the end of the interview, as if rejecting Sally's clinical terms, although Penny knew well what they meant, she said to Sally, "I just want to make sure she's going to be treated like a queen. She deserves that."

Sally kept her eyes on her notes. "She will be," she said rather curtly.

Before long on that September Saturday, the cars are loaded at Penny's house. I stand in the driveway, watching Mary tread carefully out the door, Jim and Sophie on either side holding Mary's hands, Mary's bright pink sweatshirt—the same one she wore on her birthday—like a blossom against the dark of the room behind. Mary steps down slowly. Penny and Deborah stand waiting at the bottom of the stairs and help Mary into a waiting car.

By noon the siblings have set up Mary's bed in her new small, single room at Allen Manor, positioned her lamps and dresser, installed its drawers, and gotten her new TV running. They hang familiar pictures on the walls.

In the hall I say to Penny, "This is an efficient operation."

"Oh, yeah. You get the five of us together, we do a lot."

Down the corridor, Mary and Sophie are sitting in a small, beige sitting room. FOX News plays on the TV. A bookcase holds board games and videos and figurines.

I sit with Mary. Sophie leaves to join Penny's problem solving: a shower chair that doesn't fit into the shower.

"What do you think?" I ask Mary, of everything, after they've gone.

"I don't know." She sighs. "I try not to think. It's better that way."

"You go with the flow."

"That's right." She grunts in her good-natured way. "That's all I *can* do."

I look at the games on the bookshelf and ask Mary if she still plays Scrabble, as Penny has mentioned.

"No, I'm past that stage. There's no one to play with, anyway."

Penny returns and hands Mary a chocolate-chip cookie wrapped in a wax-paper bag. She heads off again.

"I hear you'll be able to have as many of those as you want from the dining room," I say.

"Oh? I doubt it."

A tall, old woman walks in, using a cane. "I'm Betty."

Mary introduces herself.

"Oh! *You're* Mary. It's very convenient, where your room is. Next to the dining room. We play bingo downstairs. You should join us. There weren't many people there today. I don't know why." Betty walks on into the hall. "Nice to meet you," she calls back.

"Nice to meet you," Mary says.

Sophie returns. "Your phone is working! And your TV is on. The picture is better than on your old one."

"That'll be nice."

"I'd like to have a Scrabble game with you, later, to consecrate your new space."

"Okay."

The work is done, and everyone convenes in the common area. Mary says she's hungry. We head to the pub where Penny, Inga, and I had gone in April the previous year, on our way to visiting facilities, including this one.

During lunch, Mary says little. The siblings banter and laugh. Afterward, I drive home. Penny and Sophie bring Mary back to Allen Manor and get her settled. At the end of the day, Penny drives home alone.

A few weeks later, Penny arrives for one of her daily visits to Mary. An aide tells her that Mary is in a common room. Penny pads down the hall and peeks through a doorway. A volunteer is pounding out "God Bless America" on the piano. Mary sits in an armchair among the other residents. She has tipped her head back. She is singing with gusto, mouth well open, eyebrows raised.

Penny quietly watches, here in this strange place, spying on her mother. Mary looks happy, more engaged than Penny has seen her in a while. Penny feels "like a mom who's dropped her kid off at day care" and finds herself crying.

Months later, Mary develops an infection at the site of her old hip replacement, has surgery to repair the joint, and moves to a nursing home in a new facility. In the spring of 2012, Penny and I meet for lunch in the college's student center and catch up. We're back where we started, where we've met many times.

"She's pretty out of it now," Penny says. On a recent visit, Penny played a *Fresh Air* interview for Mary. Terry Gross spoke with Hugh Laurie, the star of *House,* the TV show that Penny and Mary had enjoyed for years—reruns of which, five years before, Mary had forgotten, first signaling her decline.

It seemed to Penny, sitting beside her mother's bed, that Mary was actively engaged by the interview. Mary kept her eyes closed, but her expression changed as the podcast progressed—her eyebrows rose and relaxed, her mouth scrunched and eased. Penny imagined that Mary was reacting thoughtfully to the interview— in a calm way. "She's still a little Buddha," Penny says.

The podcast ended, and Mary opened her eyes. "I'm back now."

"Oooh," Penny said. "I want to know where you *went*!"

Mary just grunted.

Here in the student center, sunlight pours in the big windows. It is a windy, bright day. Penny pulls out her computer tablet. "You want to hear my favorite Paul Simon song?"

"Yeah," I say.

Penny taps the screen, and "The Afterlife" begins—a sliding, shuffling, groovy song about getting into heaven. She sings along and totters in her chair in time to the beat, hands clenched at her sides, elbows bent and tucked. Her sister Sophie recently made up this side-to-side jiggle, Penny says. Penny likes it because it reminds her of the movements of old people—small, contained, restricted. For the chorus, Sophie has invented hand gestures, and Penny performs them now, her eyes alight with amuse-ment and a kind of joy. Simon sings, "You got to fill out a form first"—and Penny writes in the air, filling out a form for getting into heaven. In her case, it is probably also an application to a nursing home. Simon sings, "and then you wait in a line"— and Penny points out an imaginary line of people waiting at the pearly gates—or the doctor's office, surely. She waggles her fin-ger in time to the music and gestures off to the side, a Motown backup singer.

She has more time to herself. She finds herself thinking more about men in her life, and who might be available. She works after hours when she wants to. Still, her caregiving has simply changed, not ceased. While she no longer has to clean up after her moth-er's accidents, nor administer meds, nor cook Mary meals, Penny is still a fierce care manager and patient advocate. She checks in,

finds problems, speaks up to staff, sends e-mails with unambigu-
ous requests and concerns. She still plays the "smart-ass."

Being this sort of empty nester has required adjustment. Penny
finds it difficult to stay motivated on her own behalf, to care about
cooking healthy food, and to keep her house as clean and tidy as
she did when Mary lived with her. She feels lonely sometimes.
Still, she says, the new arrangement is going to work out fine: "I
think *I'm* going to be fine," with "lots of people cheering me on."

Other group members' stories evolve, too, and in some ways resolve.

Miriam talks at meetings about her new community organizing. Not long after the death of her husband, James, of Parkinson's
back in 2009, Miriam had an "epiphany." She was in the hospital,
recovering from one of her strokes. Lying in bed, she reflected on
the eleven years of grueling care for James. She had no family now,
but felt cared for by the hospital. She told one of the staff that she
wanted to do something to help others through their own caregiving exhaustion and stress. She would build on her grief by helping
other dementia caregivers.

"The next thing I knew," Miriam says, the hospital's CEO and
its chief operating officer were walking into Miriam's small hospital room. They already knew Miriam. They took seats. Looking
back, Miriam wonders how she looked: "I had spaghetti for hair.
I *hope* that the johnny I was wearing was closed in the back." She
told the administrators that she had an idea, still vague, for a center
to support caregivers and dementia patients. "Because nobody can
do this," she said, meaning give long-term care alone. "This is not
doable." The hospital's chief operating officer, Miriam says, "had
a yellow pad on her lap. She handed it to me in the bed. She said,
'Start writing.'"

Miriam worked on her vision over months. She describes it to the group. She will organize a resource center in the hospital for people with dementia and their caregivers, a place offering information and services. The center will coordinate care, help caregivers feel less alone, and abate the stigma of dementia. It will provide programs that enrich dementia patients' lives through "art, music, movement, and touch." These are "modalities that bypass intellectual skills and tap into neuropathways that *are* functioning and that *can* function," Miriam says. The approach will enhance dementia patients' mood with fewer, or without, drugs. "The goal is to improve quality of life, even as the degenerative disease is doing its number." Miriam has held meetings with doctors, nurses, social workers, artists—and generated ideas about supporting and nurturing people with dementia, and their caregivers, as they cope with change. With the right resources, the right community support, Miriam says, "Quality of life for patient—and caregiver—*will* go up."

Listening to Miriam's plans, group members nod and murmur in approval.

After years of sleep deprivation, and a growing recognition that she can no longer care for her husband, David, at home, Linda will move him to the veterans facility where Liz's husband, Joe, lives. She feels tremendous guilt and loss during this wrenching transition. Learning to live alone, after sixty-five years of marriage, requires a great shift of mind. During the first two nights by herself, she tells the group, she reached across the bed in her half sleep, searching in vain for Dave.

By the third night, though, for the first time in six years, she slept deeply for eight straight hours.

• • •

Karen's Don is diagnosed with pancreatic cancer. It progresses rapidly, and after a few months he dies at home, with Karen and other family at his side. Unlike others in the group after their spouse's death, Karen will never return to a meeting.

After the death of her husband, Harold, back in January, Katherine stays active, skiing and swimming and paddling her kayak. She returns to the group occasionally. She has a relationship with a new man. One new group member says, "So there *is* life after caregiving."

Joan hangs on, declining slowly. William keeps steadily caring for her.

Liz continues struggling with health problems—headaches, diverticulitis, a rare immune disorder. Eventually she stops visiting Joe at the veterans home altogether. She considers divorcing him, but decides against it. She stays on as Joe's health-care proxy; she pays his bills, gets occasional updates from staff. She keeps trying, in the group, to let go of her resentment toward her husband. She tells me that, with distance, a feeling of compassion toward Joe seems more possible. She is learning, she says, that compassion feels better, is less exhausting, than bitterness.

One day she musters her courage and trust and tells the group the full story of her marriage. She describes the verbal abuse, the names Joe called her, her fear of him. Everyone listens with empathy, and Liz's composure melts, for the first time ever in a group meeting. Ben takes the "lunky napkin container" and pushes it across the table toward Liz, just as he did for Sarah back in the spring of 2010. Sarah herself slides across the table a package of tissues, decorated with a lavender iris. "These are much softer," she says. "And they're just as thick." Liz laughs, takes one, and wipes her tears.

I'm changed, too. I'm disquieted. How could I not be, having followed along with everyone's great challenges? But I also feel braver, more prepared, aware—more compassionate, too, and open, even to what frightens me. One Sunday afternoon I join my mother— she is seventy-two, healthy, active, and sharp—at her house. A few years before, my mother had named me as her health-care proxy. We sit now, sock-footed, on the couch in her study, drink tea, and begin a conversation that I hope will continue for years. I say that I'd like, simply, to know what she thinks about when she thinks of getting older. She answers that she feels, as her own mother did, a strong aversion to ending up in "some place for old people," sitting idle in a drab, institutional room, mostly alone. My mother muses wryly that, who knows, depending on what happens, she might find appealing her own mother's way out. But she doesn't really expect this. She does hope to live at home until the end, in her sunlit house, surrounded by her flowering plants, her beloved dogs, and the views of hills outside her windows. She has an advance directive that is clear about her desire not to receive medical treatment were she unable to live a "meaningful and cognizant life."

We speak some about Hildegard. I realize that, just by sitting and talking together in closeness, my mother and I are walking what feels like a new and lovely path, away from Hildegard's fear of intimacy and need for absolute control. Later, hugging my mom good-bye, leaving her house, driving a half hour back to mine, I feel relief and gratitude for this generational shift.

❧ Testament

In August of 2011, I go and pick up Daniel. We will drive for an hour to a Tanglewood Saturday rehearsal, the last of the season, of the BSO's annual performance of Beethoven's Ninth.

I ask how he has been. "Okay," he says soberly from the passenger seat, with a hint of forced cheer. "It's an effortful life." He pauses. "I seem," he says, as if delivering the results of a scientific experiment, "to be persevering." He spends most of his time alone, listening to music, steeped in memories, occasionally overwhelmed by them. Friends visit, take him out for lunch. Month to month, his lymphoma surges, gets treated, subsides. His doctor still tells Daniel that he'll likely die of something other than cancer. And yet, every stay of death—each time Daniel learns that the cancer is under control again—leaves him so relieved that he weeps.

We drive south, then west. A hurricane is making its way up the East Coast. Daniel has persuaded me to travel anyway. On the interstate, we see more cars moving west than east, and I wonder aloud if people are moving away from, rather than toward, the path of the hurricane. Perhaps so, Daniel says. The sky is overcast, but does not yet look threatening. Still, I carry in my mind the computer image I've checked online for the last day: an enormous, gray, ominous spiral, caught by satellite, heading up the coast. A red line shows the storm's likely path; it crosses over Daniel's and my towns. Online, in conversations, and in my mind, there's a sense of incoming danger. Daniel and I are driving in his little car, under nature's great sky.

We pull into a spot close to Tanglewood's gate. Leanne's handicapped parking pass hangs from the rearview mirror, a photo adhered to it. Her smiling face sways over the dashboard. Earlier, putting Daniel's walker into the car, I had noticed, in the backseat,

McDonald's receipts. I picked one up; it was for a breakfast biscuit, dated a few days before Leanne committed suicide. She must have gone out to the drive-through, perhaps for the last time.

I turn off the car, and Daniel leans his thin frame over his lap. He takes a deep breath and lets out a small, voiceless sob.

We sit for a long moment. The sky is gray, the air heavy and damp. White pines grow tall on the grounds nearby. A wooded hill beyond the parking lot is dark against the gray sky.

"I can't believe I'm here," Daniel says—a statement at once full of grief, relief, and joy.

He makes the slow steps toward the open-air hall. At each crack and bump, he pauses, lifts his walker, moves it forward, places it down again, and steps forward. Tanglewood began selling assigned seats this year, so we didn't have to arrive early and wait in line—a welcome convenience. Yet the new system has also dissolved something dear to Daniel, a shared experience he enjoyed for decades.

Inside the Koussevitzky Shed—with its packed-dirt floor and high, vaulted steel beams—hundreds of people mill and take their places. We sit in the fourth row, just right of the conductor's podium. Before long, Lorin Maazel, eighty-one, strides onto the stage, wearing jeans and a blue blazer. The Boston Symphony Orchestra members, in street clothes, hands on instruments, applaud him orchestra-style, pattering their feet on the stage floor. Maazel says something to the musicians and the chorus—it sounds like "Let's get this thing done"—and they laugh. The hurricane is on everyone's mind. Maazel turns quickly to the audience and says, "Excuse my back," and the audience laughs. He raises his baton; the musicians raise their instruments.

It is perhaps the most beloved piece of music ever composed— Beethoven's expression, in part, of his life trials—grief over going deaf, a grueling battle for custody of a nephew—the result of the creativity these struggles spawned. Earlier, Daniel had told me that

Beethoven had considered suicide after learning that he'd go deaf and there was no cure. But the composer realized that, through his music, he could offer something "imperishable"—Daniel's exact word. Beethoven chose to live and create. In the Heiligenstadt Testament—a letter and will that Beethoven wrote to his brothers in 1802 and kept secret until his death in 1827—Beethoven described despair, and also a kind of hope, a renewed purpose. Perhaps he felt the peace of descending fully into discouragement and choosing life. "Perhaps I shall get better, perhaps not," the thirty-two-year-old composer wrote. "I am ready." He may have given up on hope entirely and found something more enduring: a courageous opening to suffering and beauty.

The BSO plays, and in that miracle of live music, swells of sound transform and enliven everything around us. Outside, clouds hang in the sky, thick and portentous. From mere stirrings of strings, the music grows into booms of timpani and heroic melodies. Tunes first hinted at swell into bellows, the percussion pounding. A moment further and the winds sing sweetly. Late in the symphony, in the ecstatic "Ode to Joy," the chorus—a wall of men and women, dressed in bright summer colors, on bleachers behind the orchestra—stand and sing, fervently and precisely. *Alle Menschen werden Brüder!*—all men shall become brothers!

Daniel sits quietly. Occasionally he weeps.

Shortly before its end, the symphony builds into a flurry of voices, horns, percussion, and winds; it slows briefly for a last turn through bold melody, then hurries on, ending with a final, triumphant chord.

The audience stands. Daniel pushes to his feet, steadies himself briefly with a hand on the seat in front of him, and claps heartily. Maazel motions for the musicians to bow. The chorus members applaud, raising their hands toward the conductor. The audience's ovation endures.

In the quiet afterward, Daniel and I make our way out of the row. A Saturday-morning regular—the woman from last summer, who is in her seventies but looks much younger, who teaches violin in New Jersey—calls out to Daniel from an aisle to our right: "Wasn't that *wonderful*?" She lays a hand on her chest and tips her head back. "My *heart* is restored!"

"*Yes,* it was," Daniel calls, and smiles.

Five days later, Daniel joins his support group for one of the last times. In November, he will announce that he will stop coming; he feels too old to make the trip any longer. He is also, he reminds them, a caregiver no more.

Today he takes a deep breath and, in professorial tone, gives a small speech. He seems to have prepared what he'll say. He recounts the story of his journey to Tanglewood in the path of the hurricane. He speaks of the glorious performance: "They played as I've never heard this piece before. It was *tremendous*." The symphony is, he says, one of the greatest pieces of music ever written—a hymn to brotherhood, a message for our times. The musicians played with uncommon passion and mastery.

He pauses for a long moment, head bowed, composing himself. He stares at the table in front of him, then lifts his eyes and looks around the room—at new faces, and old friends: Ben, Rufus, Linda, William, Penny. They've been watching him, listening intently, as if holding their breaths. "So this will have to last me now until next summer." Daniel chuckles softly, almost apologetically. "If I'm still around by then." Penny smiles at him, affectionately, with admiration. Daniel closes his eyes, rests his hands in his lap, and bows his head.

AUTHOR'S NOTE

When she notices an uncanny coincidence, some poetic conflu-
ence of events, Penny often laughs and says, "You can't make this
stuff *up*!" Life is so uncanny, she means, that even a fiction writer
couldn't conjure it.

This book is, indeed, a work of nonfiction, the result of three
years of reporting and research. I have not made up Penny's story
or anyone else's. Many of the scenes I witnessed. Other stories and
scenes I reconstructed from the recollections of my subjects. When
possible I corroborated stories, but in an effort to maintain my
subjects' privacy (so as not to go asking around for verification),
I have largely presented facts as they were told to me, or as they
were recalled in the support group. I often asked several times for
a recounting of the same stories, as a way of verifying details. Most
of the dialogue in the support group is the product of transcribed
recordings.

To protect my subjects' privacy, I have changed their names.
(Except one: Mary, Penny's mother, asked that I use her real first
name.) I also changed the names of some places or simply refrained
from identifying them.

Throughout the book, I often describe the feelings and
thoughts of the people I write about. In each of these cases, I was
able to report on these "inner" events because a subject shared
them in a support-group meeting, or in conversation with me.

NOTES ON SOURCES
AND OTHER RESOURCES

These notes provide citations for references in this book and, in some cases, include notes on these sources. They also, in some places, include further general information and resources that I hope will be useful. For updates, please see nelllake.com.

Prologue

5 *More than a third of elderly men:* Federal Interagency Forum on Aging-Related Statistics, "Older Americans 2012: Key Indicators of Well-Being," agingstats.gov/agingstatsdotnet/Main_Site/Data/2012_Documents/Docs/EntireChartbook.pdf.

5 *More than 5 million people have Alzheimer's:* Alzheimer's Association, "2013 Alzheimer's Disease Facts and Figures," alz.org/downloads/facts_figures_2013.pdf.

5 *More than 43 million Americans:* National Alliance for Caregiving and the AARP, "Caregiving in the US: A Focused Look at Those Caring for Someone Age 50 or Older," assets.aarp.org/rgcenter/il/caregiving_09.pdf.

5 *Informal caregivers are the largest source:* Family Caregiver Alliance and the AARP, "Valuing the Invaluable: The Economic Value of Family Caregiving," aarp.org/relationships/caregiving/info-07-2011/valuing-the-invaluable.html.

6 *Caregivers in general experience greater stress:* R. Schulz and S. R. Beach,

"Caregiving as a Risk Factor for Mortality: The Caregiver Health Effects Study," *Journal of the American Medical Association* 282, no. 23 (1999). For other research into the health effects of informal caregiving, see the work of Janice Kiecolt-Glaser and Ronald Glaser, pni.osumc.edu/.

Part I: Winter: Storms

29 *The previous year, the National Alliance for Caregiving:* National Alliance for Caregiving and the AARP, "Caregiving in the US: A Focused Look at Those Caring for Someone Age 50 or Older," assets.aarp.org/rgcenter/il /caregiving_09.pdf.

37 *Joan was having a "catastrophic reaction":* A good, now-classic source for information about "difficult" behavior in dementia patients, and dementia caregiving in general, is Nancy L. Mace and Peter V. Rabins, *The 36-Hour Day: A Family Guide to Caring for Persons with Alzheimer's Disease, Related Dementing Illness, and Memory Loss in Later Life* (New York: Grand Central Publishing, 1999).

   The Alzheimer's Association's website, alz.org, and its twenty-four-hour helpline, 1-800-272-3900, are other good sources for learning about catastrophic reactions, other challenging dementia behaviors, and how to respond to them.

37 *Alzheimer's patients who are hospitalized:* T. G. Fong et al., "Adverse Outcomes After Hospitalization and Delirium in Persons with Alzheimer's Disease," *Annals of Internal Medicine* 156, no. 12 (June 19, 2012).

43 *MRSA stands for methicillin-resistant* Staphylococcus aureus: The websites for the National Institutes of Health, nih.gov, and the Centers for Disease Control, cdc.gov, provide general information about MRSA and MRSA infections.

47 *"At their outer reaches . . . shame and intimacy converge":* Wendy Lustbader, *Counting on Kindness: The Dilemmas of Dependency* (New York: Free Press, 1991), 47.

47 *Latino caregivers, for example, who make up 10 percent:* Brent T. Mausbach et al., "Ethnicity and Time to Institutionalization of Dementia Patients: A Comparison of Latina and Caucasian Female Family Caregivers," *Journal of the American Geriatrics Society* 52, no. 7 (July 2004).

47 *African-Americans (who make up 11 percent of US caregivers):* W. E.

Haley et al., "Well-Being, Appraisal, and Coping in African-American and Caucasian Dementia Caregivers: Findings from the REACH Study," *Aging & Mental Health* 8, no. 4 (July 2004).

50 *Medicine was domestic and in the hands of women:* Emily Abel, *Hearts of Wisdom: American Women Caring for Kin, 1850–1940* (Cambridge, MA: Harvard University Press, 2000), 38.

50 *In the nineteenth century, by the time women reached adulthood:* Public lecture on nineteenth-century caregiving given by Elizabeth Sharpe at Mount Holyoke College, February 28, 2012.

50 *They had a "cosmological" view of the end of life:* Thomas Cole, *The Journey of Life: A Cultural History of Aging in America* (Cambridge, MA: Cambridge University Press, 1992), xxvi.

51 *Cole cites Benjamin Franklin:* Ibid., xxiv.

51 *As Victorians "conquered" the West:* Ibid., xxix.

51 *Old age to Victorians, Cole writes:* Ibid., 91.

52 *"Stated baldly," Cole writes:* Ibid., xxx.

52 *Households mostly relied on the skills and traditional knowledge:* Paul Starr, *The Social Transformation of American Medicine: The Rise of a Sovereign Profession and the Making of a Vast Industry* (New York: HarperPerennial, 1982), 32.

52 *"Sickness and insanity, childbirth and death":* Ibid., 75.

54 *No one wrote of feeling responsible for everything:* Public lecture, Sharpe, at Mount Holyoke College. Sharpe believes the evidence is strong that real differences existed between the psychological experiences of nineteenth-century women and those of today's women—that differing reports of their caregiving experiences do represent true differences in subjective experience.

55 Cure *originally meant "care and concern,":* New Oxford American Dictionary.

69 *State policies have been influenced, too, by a 1999 decision by the US Supreme Court: Olmstead v. L.C. and E.W.*

69 *direct-care workers receive little pay and are less educated:* Dorie Seavey and Abby Marquand / Paraprofessional Healthcare Institute, "Caring in America: A Comprehensive Analysis of the Nation's Fastest-Growing Jobs: Home Health and Personal Care Aides," phinational.org/sites /phinational.org/files/clearinghouse/caringinamerica-20111212.pdf, sections 7 and 8.

69 *While advocates and many state governments are trying:* Steven Edelstein is the national policy director of the Paraprofessional Healthcare Institute, which, according to its website, "works to improve the lives of people who need home or residential care, by improving the lives of the people who provide that care." Edelstein argues that if our health-care system attracted and retained good home health workers through decent wages, conditions, and training, the system would save money. Agencies, he says, would spend less on recruitment and training of new workers, and care recipients would stay healthier, making fewer trips to the hospital; and with a well-qualified home-health-care workforce, fewer people would move into expensive institutional care.

I also found helpful to this section an interview with Im Ja Choi, a recipient of a Robert Wood Johnson Foundation Community Health Leaders Award, and founding director of Penn Asian Senior Services, a nonprofit home health-care agency in Pennsylvania.

69 *I find a passage on the website of the Family Caregiver Alliance:* Family Caregiver Alliance / National Center on Caregiving, "Health Care Reform and Family Caregivers," caregiver.org/content/pdfs/HCR%20 provisions%20for%20caregivers-2010.pdf.

The need for better care coordination, particularly with transitions from one care setting to another, is getting increasing attention from policymakers and advocates. See, for example, the United Hospital Fund of New York's "Next Step in Care" program (nextstepincare.org/) and the Campaign for Better Care (nationalpartnership.org/site/PageServer? pagename=cbc_index).

70 *Meanwhile in Washington, health-care reform has stumbled along:* My brief discussion of health-care reform stems from broadly following the news of health-care reform in various media. I found useful, for general background, Starr's *Social Transformation of American Medicine*; Jonathan Cohn, *Sick: The Untold Story of America's Health Care Crisis—and the People Who Pay the Price* (New York: HarperPerennial, 2007); and the *Frontline* documentary, "Sick Around America" (season 27, ep. 10, March 31, 2009). I was also aided by an interview with Carol Levine, director of the Families and Healthcare Project at the United Hospital Fund of New York, and the articles of Atul Gawande in the *New Yorker*.

Part II: Spring: Assisted Living

96 *Liz had "low relationship satisfaction," to use one report's language:* Pamela Lee Steadman et al., "Premorbid Relationship Satisfaction and Caregiver Burden in Dementia Caregivers," *Journal of Geriatric Psychiatry and Neurology* 20, no. 2 (June 2007).

101 *checklists on nursing-home quality that she and Penny have printed off a Medicare site:* medicare.gov/NursingHomeCompare/search.aspx ?bhcp=1.

111 *"We're going to have to file a section twelve":* malegislature.gov/Laws /GeneralLaws/PartI/TitleXVII/Chapter123/Section12.

115 *The use of psychotropic drugs—often dangerous for the elderly:* For more information about psychotropic drugs in nursing homes, see, for example:

- American Geriatrics Society, "Updated Beers Criteria for Potentially Inappropriate Medication Use in Older Adults," american geriatrics.org/health_care_professionals/clinical_practice /clinical_guidelines_recommendations/2012.
- Department of Health and Human Services, "Psychotropic Drug Use in Nursing Homes," oig.hhs.gov/oei/reports/oei-02-00 -00490.pdf.
- American Geriatrics Society, "Ten Medications Older Adults Should Avoid or Use with Caution," americangeriatrics.org/files /documents/beers/FHATipMEDS.pdf.

115 *At least one small nursing-home experiment:* Paula Span, "Clearing the Fog in Nursing Homes," *New York Times,* February 15, 2011, newoldage .blogs.nytimes.com/2011/02/15/clearing-the-fog-in-nursing-homes/.

115 *The problem, however, according to the Centers for Medicare & Medicaid Services:* Centers for Medicare & Medicaid Services' Office of Clinical Standards and Quality, "2012 Nursing Home Action Plan: Action Plan for Further Improvement of Nursing Home Quality," cms.gov /Medicare/Provider-Enrollment-and-Certification/Certificationand Complianc/Downloads/2012-Nursing-Home-Action-Plan.pdf.

118 *Sarah recommends a book:* Naomi Fell and Vicki de Klerk-Rubin, *The Validation Breakthrough: Simple Techniques for Communicating with People*

with Alzheimer's and Other Dementias, 3rd ed. (Baltimore, MD: Health Professions Press, 2012).

Part III: Summer: "Never Forget"

136 *Pauline Boss, a researcher and psychotherapist:* Pauline Boss, *Ambiguous Loss: Learning to Live with Unresolved Grief* (Cambridge, MA: Harvard University Press, 1999).

140 *Men's and women's care seem to show broad differences:* Betty J. Kramer and Edward H. Thompson Jr., eds., *Men as Caregivers* (New York: Springer Publishing, 2002). I found the chapter "Psychosocial Challenges and Rewards Experienced by Caregiving Men: A Review of the Literature and an Empirical Case Example," by Elizabeth H. Carpenter and Baila H. Miller, especially useful.

147 *People with dementia sometimes behave inappropriately:* When dementia patients' behavior becomes inappropriate, experts advise gently redirecting their attention toward other things. Avoiding situations in which the behavior is likely to arise can be helpful, too. See, for instance, *The 36-Hour Day,* cited previously.

163 *James McGaugh, eminent brain researcher:* James McGaugh, *Memory and Emotion: The Making of Lasting Memories* (New York: Columbia University Press, 2003).

171 *"So the guns have reared their ugly heads":* A tip sheet on guns and safety from the Alzheimer's Association is available online at alz.org/cacentral /documents/14-safety_and_the_right_to_bear_arms.pdf.

172 *In addition to guns, the group often discusses another danger:* I thank Nina Silverstein, professor of gerontology at the University of Massachusetts Boston, for sharing her expertise on the topic of dementia and driving, particularly for the idea that objects can "cue" problem behavior.

Driving is often one of the most difficult issues in dementia caregiving, in part because operating an automobile, Silverstein says, involves many skills beyond accelerating, braking, and turning. Before dementia patients lose these abilities, their "executive function" declines, so that the greatest danger lies in their difficulty perceiving and navigating traffic— and in the complexity of finding one's way from point A to point D.

A survey of research by the American Academy of Neurology (AAN) confirms that people with dementia, like Don, have difficulty assessing their driving ability (D. J. Iverson, G. S. Gronseth, M. A. Reger, et al., "Practice Parameter Update: Evaluation of Driving Risk in Dementia," *Neurology Journal* 74 [January 10, 2011]: 1316). In one study cited in the survey, 94 percent of a group of patients with mild Alzheimer's disease called themselves safe drivers, but only 41 percent of them passed an on-road driving test. The AAN report also discusses the issue of determining whether a dementia patient should be *allowed* to drive. The report's standards are vague, however, and leave decisions largely to clinicians' discretions. The American Association for Geriatric Psychiatry takes a slightly stronger position: "Discontinuation of driving should be strongly considered for all patients" who have been diagnosed with Alzheimer's ("AAGP Position Statement: Principles of Care for Patients with Dementia Resulting from Alzheimer Disease," gmhfonline.org /prof/position_caredmnalz.asp).

Many laypeople lean on a more folksy standard: if you are afraid to be driven by a person with dementia, or if you wouldn't want him or her to drive your children, or if you're worried about the safety of someone in a crosswalk in front of the driver—he or she should be asked to give up the keys.

This is the trickiest matter of all. Advice from dementia-advocacy and other organizations—and from caregivers who have been through the difficulty—includes: Ask a doctor to play the "bad guy" by writing a "prescription" not to drive. Start the conversation about driving as soon as memory loss is recognized. Help the person with dementia find transportation alternatives. In videos on the Alzheimer's Association website, actors demonstrate interactions between caregivers and care recipients.

For more information and/or help with the issue of dementia and driving see, for example:

- The Alzheimer's Association's online guide to the issue of driving and dementia, which includes the videos mentioned above: alz .org/care/alzheimers-dementia-and-driving.asp.
- The American Occupational Therapy Association Inc. can help with finding a therapist to do a driving assessment: myaota.aota .org/driver_search/index.aspx.
- ITN America is a nonprofit organization that works to provide

"sustainable, community-based transportation services" to the elderly: itnamerica.org.

181 *"Have you hit the brick wall?":* This seems a good place to offer a few resources that may help with the building stress of long-term caregiving:

- Department of Health and Human Services. At eldercare.gov, find out which agencies in your area assist with locating services such as adult day care, home health care, and caregiver training and education. At longtermcare.gov find information on Medicare and Medicaid and other resources that help with planning for long-term care. The Alzheimer's Association, alz.org or 1-800-272-3900, provides information, support, and help finding an Alzheimer's support group.
- AARP. Part of the AARP's website is aimed at supporting caregivers (aarp.org/home-family/caregiving/). The AARP site also provides a booklet that helps caregivers plan (aarp.org/home-family/care giving/info-07-2012/prepare-to-care-planning-guide.html), and a caregiving support line (1-888-333-5885).
- The Family Caregiver Alliance's website, caregiver.org, provides opportunities to share experiences and offers information, as does caregiving.com.
- The Rosalynn Carter Institute for Caregiving's website includes a comprehensive list of resources for caregivers of all sorts: rosalynn carter.org/caregiver_resources/.

Part IV: Fall and Early Winter: The Far Shore

194 *"Life is pleasant. Death is peaceful":* Isaac Asimov, *Fantastic Voyage II: Destination Brain* (London: Grafton, 1988), 96.

194 *"We rarely go gentle into that good night":* Sherwin Nuland, *How We Die: Reflections on Life's Final Chapter* (New York: Alfred A. Knopf, 1993), 9.

199 *This helps explain an undercounting of Alzheimer's deaths:* Alzheimer's Association, "Alzheimer's Disease Facts and Figures," alz.org/downloads /facts_figures_2013.pdf, 24.

200 *Studies show that opting only for comfort care:* Jennifer S. Temel et al.,

"Early Palliative Care for Patients with Metastatic Non-Small-Cell Lung Cancer," *New England Journal of Medicine* 363, no. 8 (August 19, 2010).

For an insightful look at palliative care, see Atul Gawande, "Letting Go: What Should Medicine Do When It Can't Save Your Life?" *New Yorker,* August 2, 2010.

205 *Survivors face much higher risk of trauma:* Alexi A. Wright et al. "Place of Death: Correlations with Quality of Life of Patients with Cancer and Predictors of Bereaved Caregivers' Mental Health," *Journal of Clinical Oncology* 28 (October 10, 2010).

221 *She says she has heard that caregivers:* Caring for a chronically ill family member does increase one's risk of death. A study in the *Journal of the American Medical Association* found that caregivers had a 63 percent higher risk of death than noncaregiving counterparts (R. Schulz and S. R. Beach, "Caregiving as a Risk Factor for Mortality: The Caregiver Health Effects Study," *Journal of the American Medical Association* 282, no. 23 [1999]).

Other work by researchers at Ohio State University found that the stress of caregiving increases inflammation, causes cells to age faster, and diminishes immune response (see the studies of Drs. Janice Kiecolt-Glaser and Ronald Glaser, pni.osumc.edu). Much research has also found that caregiving is associated with higher rates of depression and anxiety.

Part V: Another Year Unfolds

251 *One in three adults aged sixty-five or older falls:* Centers for Disease Control, cdc.gov/HomeandRecreationalSafety/Falls, and National Council on Aging, ncoa.org/improve-health/falls-prevention.

283 *She will organize a resource center in the hospital:* Miriam's envisioned resource center would seek to ease the problems of access and coordination for dementia caregivers, particularly those who have their loved ones at home. A big challenge in keeping dementia patients at home is that caregivers must often find and continually coordinate disparate, fragmented resources—such as adult day care, home health aides, caregiving support, and training.

The new approach to dementia care that Miriam hopes to advance in her community is slowly gaining hold nationwide. The strategy seeks to minimize the use of psychotropic drugs and focuses on reducing patients' pain and stress while enhancing their enjoyment and self-expression. It uses therapy techniques such as drawing, massage, music, and writing. It also strives to engage dementia patients in activities they enjoyed in the past, seeks to create soothing environments, and promotes exercise.

Research backs up the idea that people with dementia benefit from approaches that seek to soothe, calm, and satisfy emotional needs. One study showed that in people with memory disorders, positive emotions after pleasant experiences lingered, even when the original experience had been forgotten (Justin S. Feinstein, Melissa C. Duff, and Daniel Tranel, "Sustained Experience of Emotion After Loss of Memory in Patients with Amnesia," *Proceedings of the National Academy of Sciences of the United States of America* 107, no. 17 [April 27, 2010]). Another study showed that a low frequency of enjoyable activities increased depression and anxiety in Alzheimer's patients (Rebecca G. Logsdon and Linda Teri, "The Pleasant Events Schedule-AD: Psychometric Properties and Relationship to Depression and Cognition in Alzheimer's Disease Patients," *Gerontologist* 37, no. 1 [1997]).

285 *We sit now, sock-footed, on the couch:* A good resource for learning about, and finding encouragement to have, conversations with loved ones about their end-of-life wishes is the Conversation Project, theconversation project.org.

288 *"Perhaps I shall get better, perhaps not,":* Barry Cooper et al., *The Beethoven Compendium: A Guide to Beethoven's Life and Music* (London: Thames and Hudson, 1991), 170.

ACKNOWLEDGMENTS

Heartfelt gratitude, first, to the caregivers: Penny, Daniel, William, Liz, Inga, Sarah, Karen, Claire, Miriam, Linda, Katherine, Carolyn. Thank you for your trust, openness, humor, and courage. I learned much from you. Thank you, Ben, for inviting me to the group. Thank you also to Mary, Joan, Joe, Don, David, Walter, Rachel, for allowing me into your lives.

Enormous thanks to Mark Kramer, my longtime friend and teacher. This book's voice, structure, and themes have been deeply informed by Mark's exquisite skill and insight. Big thanks, also, to the members of Mark's writing workshop, convened in his kitchen—including, over the years, Catherine Buni, Marc Chalufour, Jim Collins, Michael Fitzpatrick, Daniel Grossman, Susan Kaplan, Paul Kramer, Kristen Laine, Jon Palfreman, Farah Stockman, Karen Weintraub, Robert Weiss, and Christine Woodside.

Thank you to my near-and-far girlfriends and their families for helping make this life of mothering and work so meaningful and fun: Sarah Buttenwieser, Kara Chapdelaine, Leslie Charles, Nan Childs, Kirsten Cirincione, Anni Crofut, Kathy Elsea, Naira Francis, Liz Friedman and my friends in her Motherwoman group, Ruth von Goeler, Jennifer Gottlieb, Ellen Kiron, Gabriella Moller, Melissa Nebelski, Katherine Nguyenle, Paula Nieman, Stephanie Pasternak, Andrea Porter, Sarah Rossmassler, Laurie Sanders, Sarah Swersey, Heather Warner, Anne Werry, Sienna Wildfield.

As a mother who craved space and time to write, I am grateful to the Turkey Land Cove Foundation, especially Kitty Burke and Emily Levett, for ten priceless days of solitude and writing on Martha's Vineyard. Thanks to Wil Hastings for critical writing time at his condominium. Thanks to the Writers' Mill.

Thank you, Richard Todd, Stephanie Soscia, Katharine Whittemore, Karen Weintraub (again), and Catherine Buni (again) for important and insightful late-draft readings. Thank you, Daniel Okrent and Susan Todd, for support in various forms.

Enormous thanks to Geri Thoma, my agent, who took on my book proposal and worked her magic with exceptional grace and kindness and skill; to Alexis Gargagliano, my first editor at Scribner, who believed in the book; and to Whitney Frick, my second editor, who jumped in with enthusiasm and applied keen discernment toward making it better. Thanks, also, to copyeditor Steve Boldt, to Daniel Burgess, and the others at Scribner who help turn manuscripts into books.

Thank you, Julie Katzman, for your warm encouragement; Robert Winsor and Valerie Yockey, Drew Winsor, Amanda Rose—and many other Winsors—for your love and kindness; Susan Crofut and Anni Crofut (again) for the chat about Hildegard; Dana Flower Lake, for your friendship; my dear siblings, Eliza Lake and Tim Lake, for sharing your expertise in long-term care and healthcare policy; my father, Anthony Lake, for a lifetime of inspiration; my mother, Antonia Lake, for the great gift of your friendship, interest, and insight.

Thank you, every day, to my boys: Douglas, for two decades of love and adventure. Galen and Jordy, I am one lucky mama. You three are my haven, my home, the light I live by.